Emotional Self-Care for Black Women

A Powerful Emotional Health Workbook to Raise Your Self-Esteem and Heal Yourself

By

Alexandra Gauff

Emotional Self-Care for Black Women: A Powerful Emotional Health Workbook to Raise Your Self-Esteem and Heal Yourself

Copyright © 2023 Alexandra Gauff

All images are courtesy of the public domain unless otherwise noted.

All rights reserved. No part of this book may be used or reproduced in any manner without written permission from the author and publisher except in the case of brief quotations embodied in critical articles or reviews.

"Self-esteem comes from being able to define the world in your own terms and refusing to abide by the judgments of others."

—Oprah Winfrey

Contents

Introduction 1

Chapter 1: Understanding Emotional Self-Care 3

Chapter 2: Components of Emotional Health 8

Chapter 3: Signs of Poor Emotional Health 24

Chapter 4: How to Improve Your Emotional Health 39

Chapter 5: The Race War 55

Chapter 6: Find Confidence in Your Blackness 67

Chapter 7: Prepare for the Road Ahead 80

Chapter 8: Build Your Self-Worth 94

Chapter 9: Prioritize Your Goals 107

Conclusion 126

Thank You 128

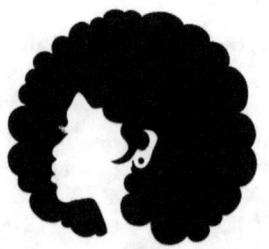

Introduction

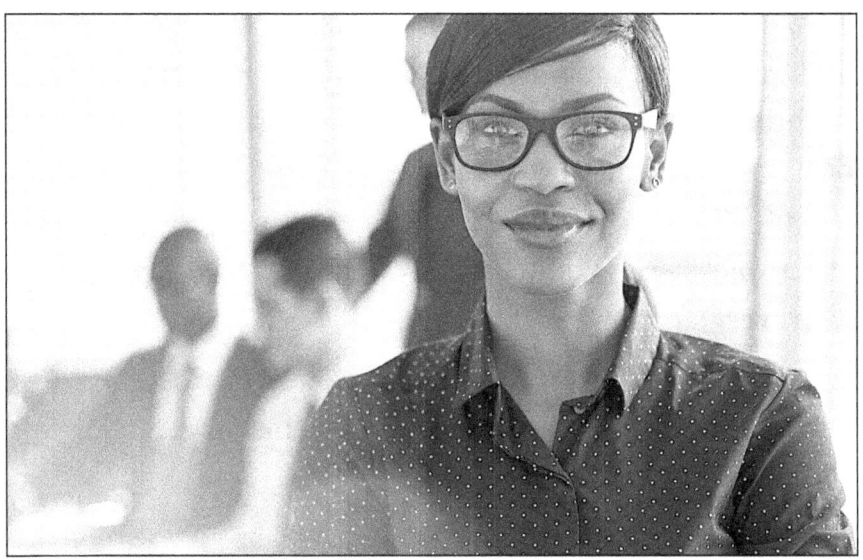

The strong black woman is a trope that has been established by an external body, inculcated into the hearts of budding young black women and ferociously espoused by them throughout the years, dating back to the era of slavery. It is no secret that women are bearers of a distinct and different strength than that of men, and it should be celebrated. But black women, in particular, have been reminded of their strength, which is usually the strength to endure the hardships of being a black body in an anti-black world, in a manner that has caused it to actually become detrimental to their emotional constitution.

Black women believe that they should be strong enough to endure the incessant hardships of life in a manner that is not promoted for alternate races. This leads to unsustainable repression of essential feelings that culminates into burnout, self-negligence, and in some cases, an acquired taste for nihilism and purposelessness. Needless to say, this book attempts to reverse the damaging effects of the strong black woman trope. It is here to remind women of their need for love, as strength without life is actually just an endurance of suffering. Black women need to start taking ownership of their own well-being in a way that seeks to preserve their inner divinity. There is nothing honorable about exuding strength when your spirit is quite literally being stripped of its vitality with every step that you take.

Emotional self-care for black women is the start of a journey toward self-recognition, which includes rest, repair, and recovery.

Black women need to remember that they are living organisms with psycho-physiological states that need to be acknowledged and treated accordingly. This is a workbook that aims to provide black women with the tools and knowledge to navigate their existence with a little bit more self-compassion, understanding, and healing.

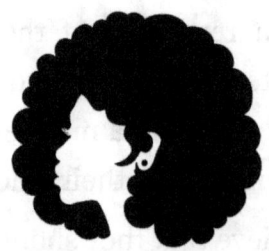

Chapter 1: Understanding Emotional Self-Care

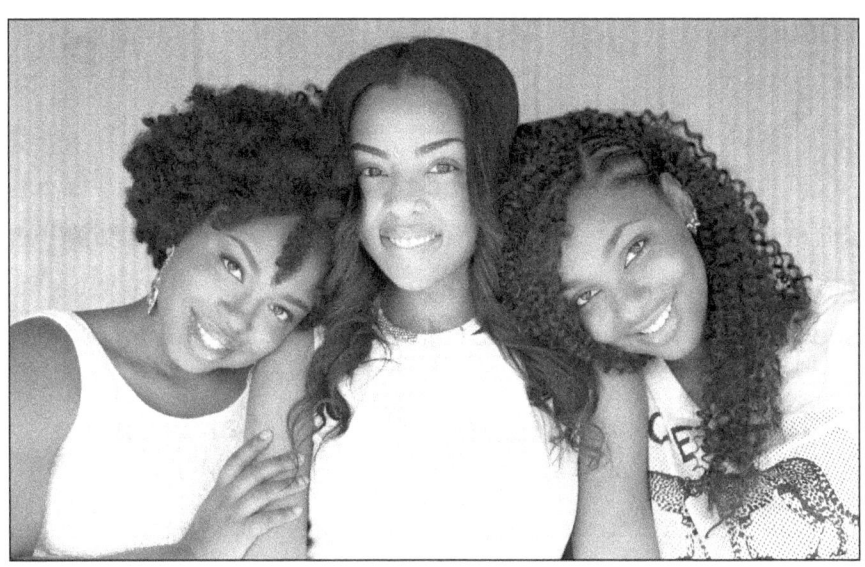

Emotional self-care can sound awfully similar to mental health care. Although both practices deal with the repair of one's intangible aspects, they are not the same.

What is the Definition of Emotional Self-Care?

The maintenance of your mental health plays a significant role in your overall health and fitness. Your emotional existence has an impact on both your physical and mental health. If you can learn to take care of your emotional needs, you will be more likely to have a happier, healthier life.

In order to practice emotional self-care, you must be able to recognize your feelings and allow yourself to express them in a way that promotes your overall well-being. You'll be better equipped to deal with the fluctuations of life when you approach your emotions and the expression thereof in a healthy way. Being emotionally disconnected increases your risk of developing stress, depression, anxiety, and other mental health problems.

Gaining a deeper awareness of your own emotions has advantages because everyone feels a vast array of distinct emotions. You may start living a healthier and happier life as soon as you begin an emotional self-care practice.

Emotional Health vs. Mental Health

Mental health and emotional health are not the same thing. Despite their connection, their meanings are extremely different. Treatments for emotional and mental health are frequently confused by people. These kinds of programs, however, are very dissimilar. Although both types of treatments address various underlying issues that might cause addictive or erratic behaviors, they essentially seek to treat slightly different states of imbalance.

Mental health is more concerned with the psychological aspects of the human psyche. Mental health treatments can affect emotional health treatments and vice versa, as emotional health seeks to deal with one's feelings. Emotional health is primarily about the feelings sparked by the data processed, whereas mental health is about how we process all the information we come across. Mental and emotional health are distinct but related. One's capacity to deal with and regulate emotions is referred to as emotional health. The capacity to form wholesome relationships is also part of it. The capacity to reason clearly and make wise decisions is a sign of mental health. It also includes the capacity to handle stress and control one's emotions. A more simplified way to view it is to consider your mental health as the hardware and your emotional health as the software. The former is primarily concerned with thinking whereas the latter is primarily concerned with feeling.

Behaviors that pertain to our brains are included in mental health domain. Mental health issues commonly arise as a result of a chemical imbalance in the brain. Some common mental health concerns are:

- depression
- anxiety
- post-traumatic stress disorder
- bipolar disorder

Several factors can cause a chemical imbalance in the brain. A natural chemical imbalance that results in a mental health problem is one of the ways in which people find themselves battling a mental illness. Usually, this issue might develop if mental illness runs in the family. However, chemical imbalances can also develop when a person uses medicines that alter their perceptual field, resulting in imbalanced hormones and the potential to develop a mental illness. On the other hand, emotional health addresses emotive issues.

Even though emotional and mental health are two distinct concepts, they are nevertheless linked. Without mental health care, people's emotions are susceptible to running dramatically out of control.

Purely concentrating on emotional well-being throws the mind off balance, making it challenging to carry out daily tasks. Although this book is about emotional health, it also seeks to further illustrate the importance of seeking out a balanced approach to health by including mental and physical health practices in one's life. At the end of the day, the human being is a web of interlinked sectors that work synergistically to produce a healthy you. An improvement or decline in one sector affects all the others.

Why is Emotional Self-Care Imperative to Your Health and Wellness?

You can feel better about yourself and be more confident when facing unforeseen circumstances by consistently tending to your emotional well-being. It might encourage adaptability, resilience, and the capacity to handle the unavoidable obstacles of life.

Neglecting one's emotional well-being can adversely affect one's mental, physical, and social well-being. When things don't go as planned, people can get overwhelmed, irritable, and unable to handle the adversities of daily life. Emotions and health have been linked. Researchers have discovered that those who linger on their negative emotions are more likely to experience a somatic manifestation of their pain, whereas people with a more upbeat positive perspective on life are generally healthier and live longer.

If people don't take care of their emotional health, their bodies could suffer.

Inflammation might worsen as a result of ongoing emotional conflict brought on by unfavorable or unresolved feelings. This can eventually lead to numerous health concerns, including cardiovascular disease, metabolic problems, and some forms of cancer.

Black women who find that their emotional lives are often riddled with issues can benefit greatly from practicing emotional self-care.

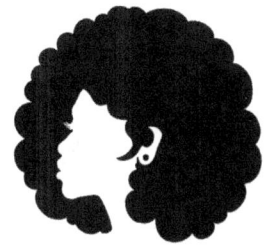

Chapter 2: Components of Emotional Health

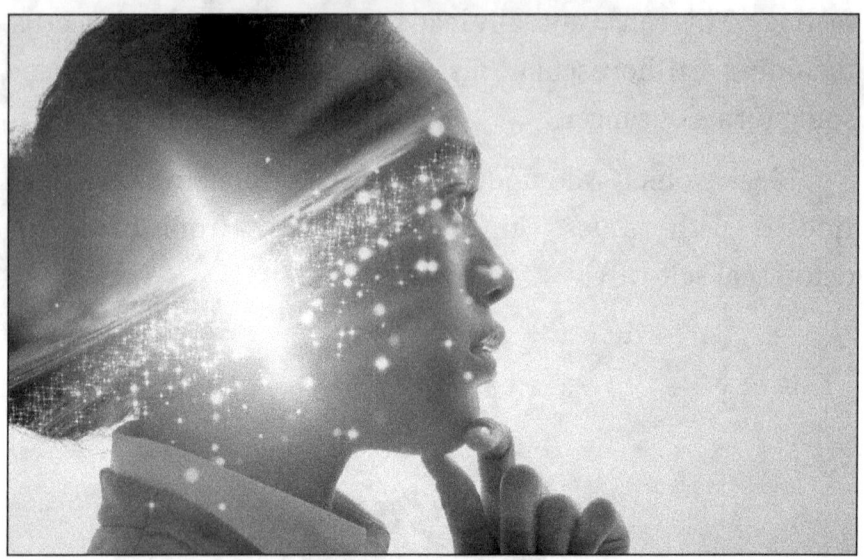

Science directed its primary concerns toward the physical body, seeking ways to heal us from our tangible ailments. Much of recent health has begun to take a closer look inward to the realms of the mind and emotions. This is where the components of emotional health reside.

Self-Awareness and Emotional Agility

Self-awareness is the capacity to focus on oneself and determine whether or not one's behaviors, ideas, or emotions are consistent with one's internal standards. You can control your emotions, match your actions with your ideals, and accurately assess how other people see you if you have a high level of self-awareness.

Simply put, people with high levels of self-awareness are able to analyze their behaviors, emotions, and ideas from a bird's-eye view.

It's a unique talent because many of us perceive our circumstances based solely on our emotions. Being self-aware is crucial for black women because it enables them to evaluate their progress and pitfalls to better re-orient themselves in a world that can be far too demanding and unkind to them.

There are two significant subcategories of self-awareness consistently emerging across several studies. The first, which we call internal self-awareness, refers to how clearly we understand our own values, desires, and aspirations, as well as how they fit with our surroundings and how they affect others. It also includes our thoughts, feelings, behaviors, strengths, and weaknesses. Internal self-awareness is linked negatively to anxiety, tension, and depression and positively to greater relationship and job satisfaction, social control, and happiness.

External self-awareness is the second category, and it refers to being aware of how others perceive us in light of the same aspects as those mentioned above. People are better at evoking empathy and understanding other people's viewpoints when they are aware of how others perceive them.

We can better understand our values, ideas, feelings, actions, strengths, and shortcomings by taking a close look at ourselves. We are conscious of the impact we have on other people. Those who are self-aware are happier and have stronger interpersonal interactions. Along with greater professional happiness, they also feel more in control of their personal and social lives.

We may see how others perceive us when we turn our gaze outward. People who are conscious of how others perceive them are more likely to be sympathetic toward others. Leaders are more inclined to include, empower, and recognize others if their opinion of themselves is consistent with that of others.

As we already discussed, improving self-awareness provides a number of advantages. These advantages vary depending on the person in question.

Here are a few instances of typical advantages of self-awareness:

- Empowers us to have a say in how things turn out.
- Enables us to make wiser decisions.
- Enables us to view things from a variety of angles.
- Extricates us from our biases and presumptions.
- Facilitates the development of stronger bonds between people.
- Improves our capacity to control our emotions.
- Lessens stress and uplifts our mood.

All emotions have the power to improve our capability to be dynamic and capable of handling complexity, stress, and setbacks. Fixed ideas about what constitutes "good" and "bad" emotions can make us judgmental, less compassionate toward others and ourselves, and less able to cope with the difficulties of life. On the flip side, emotional agility enables black women to process their emotions with compassion and curiosity while letting go of preconceived notions and judgments from the past.

When black women are emotionally agile, they are able to thrive in spite of their emotions rather than becoming controlled by them. The labels "good" and "bad" must be abandoned in order to embrace a whole spectrum of emotions. This will help them to develop their emotional agility.

Coping Skills

People employ coping mechanisms to deal with difficult circumstances. Effective stress management can improve their physical and mental health as well as their capacity to perform at a high level both in their personal and professional life.

Technically, getting enough sleep, eating a balanced diet, and exercising frequently are all healthy habits that lower stress. However, when we discuss coping mechanisms, we typically refer to techniques that offer greater short-term satisfaction. Coping mechanisms are actions we can take in the heat of the moment to reduce the intensity of our feelings and prevent becoming overpowered by them. A coping mechanism can assist us in navigating difficult circumstances with a bit more ease while simultaneously helping us avoid engaging in activities that are harmful or would cause shame or regret.

It is not uncommon to hear people criticizing coping mechanisms, saying that they are superficial fixes for more serious issues. They claim that coping mechanisms deal with symptoms without attempting to identify their cause. While attempting to calm herself, a black woman who employs deep breathing to control anxiety is unlikely to realize what brought on the fear in the first place.

Coping mechanisms are sometimes viewed as too superficial to bring about long-term change.

While this perspective is not erroneous per se, it does not seek to evaluate coping mechanisms for what they truly are but instead relies on a strawman argument to undermine their psychological importance. Black women can explore their problems more deeply by using their coping mechanisms as a starting point to alleviate uncomfortable feelings in the moment while simultaneously seeking to understand the root cause of said feelings. When a woman learns and uses coping mechanisms, she realizes that she can wield a certain degree of control over her emotions and the way she chooses to handle them. This sense of control can easily propel black women to new heights, as they can become inspired to make a change in other areas of their lives once they see they can, in fact, create tangible changes. However, coping mechanisms are not a panacea; they should be utilized as an alleviation method and not a cure, akin to taking painkillers when you have the flu. The painkillers alleviate short-term pain, but the flu is the real issue that needs to be addressed.

For black women with mild anxiety or life stressors, learning a few effective coping skills may be all they need to feel better. However, most black women with diagnosable mental health struggles, like anxiety or depression, will need therapy beyond coping skills in order to heal. Finding coping skills that work well can lay a strong foundation for future therapy. The coping mechanisms used by black women may be influenced by the junction of their racial and gender identities.

Race, socioeconomic status, and gender must be taken into account as stressors and as influences on the coping mechanisms used by this demographic. Participants in qualitative research on black women's coping strategies noted a wide range of stressors, including juggling several responsibilities, having to take care of others, and serving as family members' "go-to person." A vast range of these stressors might be indications of black women's efforts to conform to the strong black woman stereotype. In order to deal with these stressors, black women used both types of coping mechanisms, namely emotion-focused and problem-focused.

Emotion-focused coping aims to lessen the unfavorable emotional reactions brought on by stress. When the cause of stress is something that the person cannot control, emotion-focused therapies may be their only viable alternative. These methods are usually:

- distractions such as keeping busy to divert your attention from the problem
- emotional openness entails expressing intense feelings by speaking or writing
- praying for wisdom and courage
- mindfulness meditation
- eating extra comfort food
- consuming alcohol
- drug abuse
- suppressing unfavorable feelings or thoughts
- long-term suppression of emotions impairs immunological functions and negatively impacts physical health.

Problem-focused coping served as a barrier between depression symptoms and discrimination. Problem-focused coping reduced the strength of the association between depression and discrimination, but avoidant coping increased that association. These results imply that for black women, problem-focused coping may be more adaptive. Researchers looked at whether the link between gendered racism and psychological suffering was mediated by an Afro-cultural coping strategy. They discovered that the positive association between gendered racism and psychological discomfort was partially mediated by cognitive-emotional coping, which is akin to avoidant coping. Therefore, black women may experience more distress while using avoidant coping mechanisms. Examples of problem-focused coping mechanisms are:

- asking a friend or a qualified individual for assistance
- establishing a to-do list
- solving problems by yourself
- setting up clear boundaries
- leaving stressful situations by walking away from them
- improving your time management

In general, problem-focused coping is the best since it eliminates the stressor, addresses the problem's underlying causes, and offers a long-term solution. Discrimination, HIV infections, and diabetes are a few examples of stresses that can be successfully managed using problem-focused solutions.

However, employing problem-focused techniques isn't always feasible. For instance, these techniques may not benefit the bereaved when someone passes away.

Emotionally focused coping is necessary for overcoming the sense of loss. Additionally, researchers have particularly taken into account how work-related stress differs from general stress. Black women are expected to successfully juggle obligations to their profession, their family, and the community at large. This situation is exacerbated by the superwoman syndrome that black women are expected to abide by. In a study, it was discovered that participants most frequently cited coping mechanism was spirituality. Both problem-focused and emotion-focused coping strategies were mentioned by the participants. However, emotion-focused coping was employed more frequently. In the past, studies have shown that black women often use spirituality as a coping mechanism in their lives. Whether this is through traditional religion—usually Christianity—or unorthodox or ancestral spiritual practices, it still serves as a powerful mechanism to abate some of the negative emotions felt by this demographic.

Spirituality has been cited by black women as having a variety of coping mechanisms, including protection, a source of inner strength, general guidance, decision-making support, and the ability to reassess pressures. More studies have backed up black women's use of spirituality as a stress-reduction strategy.

Black women claimed to rely on their beliefs, turn to their ancestors for help, value themselves, and value others. These findings confirm earlier research findings that black women frequently seek social support and turn to spirituality or religion as a coping mechanism.

Black women reacted to gendered racism by relying on others or transforming into superwomen. The stereotype of the strong black woman may allow them to demonstrate their accomplishments to others and shield themselves from the repercussions of gendered discrimination. Black women may also utilize escape as a coping mechanism or avoidance techniques like eating or napping. Black women employ a variety of coping mechanisms to deal with different sorts of oppression.

In addition to looking at the particular coping mechanisms employed by black women, academics have examined how different coping mechanisms and distress relate to one another. According to the efficiency of coping theory, adaptive coping lessens suffering, whereas maladaptive coping worsens it. Unfortunately, black women endure sexism, racism, and gendered racism on a daily basis. Therefore, the coping mechanisms used as a response to these oppressive forms may either lessen or increase psychological suffering. To explore how black women deal with racism, a framework of avoidant-focused and problem-focused coping methods were applied.

Living with Purpose

Psychologists have been researching how lifelong, significant goals emerge for decades. Launching a business, studying an illness, or teaching children to read are examples of objectives that have the potential to improve the lives of others.

In fact, a feeling of purpose seems to have developed in humans so that we might do great things together, which may explain why it is linked to improved mental and physical health. In this way, the purpose seems to be an adaptive mechanism of evolution. It promotes the survival of both the individual and the entire species.

Many people appear to believe that your unique talents and ability to stand out from the crowd give you a sense of purpose, but that is only partially true. A crisis of purpose is frequently a sign of isolation because it also develops from our lack of connection to others. When you find your way, you'll certainly run into other people who are also seeking the same thing: a sense of community.

Essentially, purpose can be described as one or more consistent and major life goals that are: deliberately chosen, arise from one's particular strengths and interests, produce future goals that direct the individual's daily actions, are intrinsically meaningful while simultaneously facilitating one's connection to someone or something outside the self. Thus, your personal, genuine set of life goals that direct your conduct, push you toward the future, and provide your life meaning are your purpose.

It's essential to understand how the concept of purpose links to meaning and values before addressing its advantages and how to define your own purpose. Purpose is frequently used interchangeably with meaning or is regarded as a component of meaning. When these two concepts are distinguished, purpose is more frequently employed to describe how a person relates the present to the future; this is because purpose is more likely to be motivating and action-oriented.

On the other hand, meaning is more about coherence and cognitive connections, particularly those that link the present to the past. One gets the impression that life has meaning from it. Even with these clear demarcations, it is possible that there is a strong reciprocal relationship between these two concepts; purpose can be influenced by experiencing meaning, and meaning can be found through seeking purpose.

A person's values in life are directly tied to their sense of purpose. Values refer to our preferences for interacting with external reality, other people, and ourselves in particular ways. Values are the principles we want to live by, the behaviors we want to adopt, the types of people we want to be, and the strengths and character traits we want to cultivate.

A strong sense of direction in life is priceless. Famous psychiatrist and concentration camp survivor Viktor Frankl stressed how having a sense of purpose may help people go through even the most trying and depressing situations. In *Man's Search for Meaning*, published in 1946, he described life in Nazi Auschwitz, demonstrating the veracity of Nietzsche's statement that "he, who has a "why" to live for, can bear with almost any how." The awareness that one's existence has a purpose is sufficient for people to persevere through the vicissitudes of life.

People frequently express a desire to discover their purpose, as if it were buried or hidden somewhere and all they needed to do was keep searching and digging. Purpose is more of a creation than a discovery, much like our personal happiness and well-being.

Understanding the "search" for purpose as a process of generating, selecting, or defining our own purpose, in my opinion, is the most beneficial. In the end, people must realize they are the ones being asked, not the significance of their lives. In other words, each person is asked a question by life, and they can only respond by taking responsibility for their own lives.

This means that we develop meaning and purpose through our own deeds and intentions. The external manifestation of our fundamental desires is what we refer to as purpose. Our deepest aspirations lead to purpose. If there is any discovery of a life's purpose, it merely entails the process of articulating our deepest wants in order to consistently match our actions and objectives with them. Here are three ways that you can begin to cultivate your purpose as a black woman:

Recognize How Life Ought to Feel

Doing what is important to you and consistent with your beliefs and values is at the crux of living in purpose. You will know you are living in your purpose because you can feel it. Everything is gray and lifeless when you aren't acting in accordance with your true self. You can feel the constant exhaustion or simply being excessively busy and bored. Your higher self will send you nudges or even a slap in the face to gain your attention if you consistently disregard it. Life is right when you're in alignment. Everything just works, and things are simple. You experience enthusiasm, light, and a deep appreciation for being here. You don't worry about how to get there since you are confident in yourself and enjoying the journey.

Discover Your Inner Calling

Stop looking outside of yourself for solutions. Black women have been expected to conduct themselves in a particular way, but they don't have to subscribe to modes of being that do not serve them. There is only this one life, so live it in the best way that you know how. Finding your calling may sound daunting, but the truth is that you already know what it is. Your calling is that which lights your soul on fire when you are doing it. All you have to do is pay attention. Sometimes it's crucial that we let go of the expectations that others have set for us and we learn how to listen to the voice of our internal compass to carry us through life. However, perplexity can occasionally obstruct your ability to access your soul, especially if you've been ignoring it for a while. Ask yourself what you need to learn and truly listen for the answer. Journaling is a wonderful way to help you connect with yourself and tune in to what's hidden within you.

Believe in Yourself and Disregard What Others May Think

Before we are taught the rules of life, we harbor an innate sense of perception. To live, however, is not a matter of right or wrong. No one has the right to tell you how to conduct yourself if you aren't functioning on your intuition's terms. There is always a different way to do something, and the path most trodden is not synonymous with the right path.

Visionaries are named so because they stand out as a consequence of their unconventional approaches to life. They challenge the status quo in search of what is best for them. The first step to doing what you want—even if the world seems to be against it—is to believe in yourself. Self-belief and confidence are essential. Recognize that you are the best judge of what is best for you.

Stress Level Management

Stress is a natural part of life and can spur you on to action. Even high levels of stress can be a normal part of life in the wake of a traumatic incident or a serious illness. It's normal for you to feel depressed or anxious for a period of time. However, stress experienced for a long period of time can be extremely corrosive to the mind and body. You can take steps to reduce your stress before it becomes overwhelming by learning certain techniques. Here are some general ways that you can seek to manage stress:

- Maintain a positive outlook on life.
- Recognize that some things are beyond your control.
- Instead of being aggressive, be assertive. Instead of being defensive, passive or angry, learn how to express yourself in an effective manner.
- Improve your time management skills.
- Set reasonable boundaries and decline requests that would put too much stress on your life.
- Make time for your interests and hobbies.

- Avoid using drugs, alcohol, or compulsive habits as a way to cope with stress. Alcohol and drug use might cause your body even more stress.
- Seek help from a trusted loved one or, in more severe cases, a professional.

Stress is usually caused by mental strain, but it has a very real somatic manifestation. The great thing is that you can combat stress or at least minimize its propensity to consume you and lead to more serious illnesses in the long run.

Exercise

To begin with, exercise can help you sleep better. Improved stress management also results from better sleep. People who exercise more frequently tend to obtain better deep sleep, which helps regenerate the brain and body, but doctors are not yet sure why. Just be careful not to exercise too close to bedtime, as this can disturb your sleep. Your mood will seem to benefit from exercise as well. The body releases endorphins primarily through aerobic activity. Endorphins are a feel-good hormone that can help to ease the uncomfortable feelings of stress in your body.

Diet

Eating healthy foods has advantages for your mental health in addition to your waistline. A nutritious diet can boost your immune system, balance your mood, lower your blood pressure, and lessen the negative effects of stress.

The opposite outcome may occur if there is a lot of added sugar and fat in your diet. Junk food may seem much more attractive when you are stressed, but it is probably what you should stay away from. Look for complex carbs, healthy fats, and lean proteins for a nutrient-dense and balanced diet. Antioxidants also combat stress. They safeguard your cells from the harm that ongoing stress may bring about. They are present in a plethora of foods, including beans, berries, spices, and vegetables.

Sleep

Stress can easily disrupt one's sleep. It is not uncommon to experience insomnia, which is the inability to fall asleep and stay asleep and is diagnosed as such if it occurs three times per week for at least three months. You can experience a cycle of tension and sleeplessness if you don't get enough sleep.

Sufficient and quality sleep is crucial to keep your health and stress levels in check. This pertains to both your daily schedule and the arrangement of your bedroom. The following behaviors could be helpful:

- Exercise regularly.
- Step outside in the sunshine.
- Nearing bedtime, limit your coffee and alcohol intake.
- Plan your sleeping hours.
- Avoid using gadgets 30 to 60 minutes before going to bed.
- Before going to bed, try relaxing techniques like meditation.

Chapter 3: Signs of Poor Emotional Health

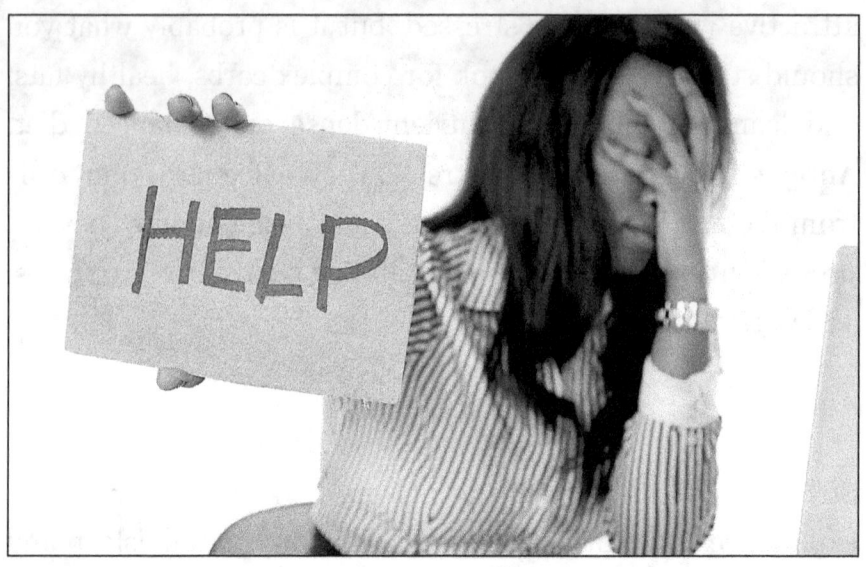

Being conscious of your feelings, thoughts, and behaviors are the first step toward having good emotional health. It's natural to develop coping mechanisms for stress and issues as you go through life. Your emotional well-being can be affected by a variety of life events. Strong emotions such as melancholy, worry, or anxiety may result from these dramatic life events and eventually lead to poor emotional health. Here are some of the signs of a person experiencing a decreased sense of emotional well-being.

Constant Exhaustion

Emotional exhaustion is the result of cumulative stress from your professional or personal life or a combination of the two.

Emotional exhaustion is one of the clear indications of burnout. People who are emotionally exhausted frequently believe they have no influence or control over life's events. They tend to feel stuck or trapped in a situation. It may be challenging to overcome emotional exhaustion if you are lacking in energy, getting inadequate sleep, or losing enthusiasm for your life. This constant state of tension has the ability to permanently harm your health over time.

Although everyone's experience of emotional tiredness is unique, common signs include the following:
- lack of motivation
- difficulty sleeping
- agitation
- feeling lethargic
- absentmindedness
- apathy
- headaches
- altered appetite
- anxiety
- depression
- difficulty concentrating
- sporadic bouts of anger
- increase in cynicism or pessimism

There is a plethora of things that can lead to emotional exhaustion over time. These could be:
- paying for an extensive education, such as medical school
- long hours at a job you despise

- having a baby
- raising children
- high-pressure positions like doctors, nurses, and police officers
- financial difficulties
- divorce proceedings
- caregiver for a chronically ill family member
- death of a friend or family member who had a long-term ailment or illness

Black women, in particular, are more predisposed to emotional exhaustion in the context of the strong black woman trope. They usually suffer in silence as they try to portray an unwavering sense of strength to the outside world while their inner reality suffers. According to a recent study, frequent or extended stress, such as that brought on by poverty or the need to show one's value in a hostile workplace, causes black women to age biologically more quickly. Microaggressions, a lack of opportunity, and the pressure to always be on the go are problems that black women commonly face. Burnout becomes nearly unavoidable when long hours, inability to log off from your e-mail, expectations of working overtime, and constant hustle mentality leave this demographic worn out and depleted.

Too Much or Too Little Sleep

Sleep quality and emotional health are closely related. Sleep quality can be impacted by having a mental health condition, and inadequate sleep can have a detrimental effect on your emotional health. So, there is a very strong link between sleep and wellness. Experts acknowledge that sleep is possibly the most crucial aspect of maintaining emotional regulation. Lack of sleep affects our capacity to control our emotions. This might eventually make us more likely to experience mental illness. As a result, illnesses like depression and anxiety may further impair sleep.

Let's start by discussing what oversleeping entails. Eight hours of sleep have long been regarded as the gold standard of sleep quantity. The National Sleep Foundation's specialists have recently reviewed recent studies to augment the sleep range to accommodate the variability of individuals. The majority of persons between the ages of 18 and 64 are said to require between seven and nine hours of sleep per night to be healthy and normal. The lowest mortality and morbidity is within seven hours, and a timeframe closer to seven hours may even be preferable, as seven hours of sleep has been associated with increased longevity and improved mental health.

More, and more, evidence suggests that sleeping too much has adverse health effects. Oversleeping appears to have a direct impact on some risk factors in some ways, but it can also be a sign of other medical problems. The proper amount of sleep varies from person to person, as some people are able to function optimally on seven hours of sleep while others may require a bit more. However, studies and experts generally agree that individuals should not sleep for longer than nine hours every night.

If you find that you consistently need more than nine hours of sleep, then you may be suffering from poor emotional health.

There has been a troubled and lengthy relationship between black people and sleep. The concept of laziness which has been used to oppress black people for centuries, is linked to the deep-seated fear of sleep in our culture. Black people currently literally cannot sleep due to years of psychological and administrative violence.

The disparities in sleep patterns between races are primarily related to socioeconomic factors as opposed to biological reasons. For instance, people who have to work two jobs are prone to sleep less than their single-occupation counterparts. This isn't always the case, as there are incredibly wealthy people who cannot afford to sleep much due to the demands of their work. Still, when observing this notion alongside racial connotations, it becomes evident that a lack of sleep permeates among the lower classes, which tend to be black people.

African Americans sleep significantly less than white people, which has a negative impact on their health. In big cities like New York, you can see this plainly when riding the subway late at night. Hispanic and black people are the ones that predominately occupy seats of empty subway cars. Their eyes flutter in an attempt to keep awake as they return to their homes after finishing their shifts. Black women in America do poorly when race, gender, and sleep are combined. They sleep 45 minutes less compared to white people and are far more prone to experience insomnia. They are more likely to go undiagnosed than white women, which makes them vulnerable to a variety of chronic illnesses.

As previously stated, a lack of sleep may be caused by societal factors, but it could also just be a result of poor emotional health. The mind incessantly runs, leaving the body to overproduce cortisol (also known as the stress hormone) which directly conflicts with the production of melatonin—the sleep hormone. A consistent cycle of this leads to chronic insomnia, which results in a cascade of other issues.

Too Much or Too Little Food

Eating habits frequently deteriorate in quality when you are experiencing a period of poor mental health. Some people eat too much and put on weight because they use food to alleviate their negative emotions. In contrast, others discover they have completely lost their appetite or are too tired to make the concerted effort toward ensuring that they are eating healthy meals.

We don't always eat to merely satiate our physical appetite. Many of us use food as a form of comfort, a way to decompress, or as a reward for ourselves. When we do eat for emotional purposes, we frequently turn to sugary snacks, fast food, and other comforting but equally harmful foods. When you're feeling low, your food cravings are rarely a plate of broccoli. Instead, you will most likely reach for a pint of ice cream, order a pizza out of boredom or loneliness, or stop at the drive-through for an extra-large milkshake after a trying day at the office.

Emotional eating is the practice of consuming food to satisfy emotional rather than actual hunger. Although there is a dopaminergic effect of food, and a momentary relief of emotional eating doesn't address emotional issues. In reality, it typically worsens your mood. The initial emotional problem persists thereafter, and you have the additional guilt feeling that comes with having overindulged in a food item for the wrong reasons.

It's not always a negative thing to use food as a reward, a pick-me-up, or for celebration purposes. However, it does become worrisome if eating is your main coping strategy when you are in emotional distress. If your first reaction is to run to the fridge anytime you're anxious, unhappy, angry, lonely, tired, or bored, you run the risk of becoming trapped in a negative cycle where the real issue or sensation is never addressed.

You cannot satiate your emotional hunger with food. Even though eating is a pleasurable activity and it may feel good in the moment, the emotions that caused the cravings are still present after the food has been consumed. And instead of feeling better after consuming the food, you feel worse due to the extra and usually empty calories that you have just consumed. It is easy for you to start blaming yourself for not having the willpower to combat the negative emotional states without needing comfort foods in the process.

Another insidious effect of emotional eating is that over time, you will find it harder and harder to manage your weight due to the excess calories consumed, and the strong neurochemical pathways that have been formed due to your habitual use of food for comfort are extremely difficult to change. This can lead you to start feeling helpless in the face of both food and emotions.

Conversely, there is a different group of people who, instead of over-eating during emotional distress, do the opposite. These types of people discover that when they're feeling down, their appetite declines. They occasionally unintentionally lose weight. They begin skipping meals and lose their appetite, and can even go as far as falling asleep during meals. When they are experiencing a phase of poor mental health, they might not feel like they have the drive or energy to eat. Additionally, stress might contribute to a decrease in appetite. When you are stressed, worried, or depressed, food doesn't seem as appetizing. However, not eating enough might increase your sensitivity and irritability, which can make your depression worse.

Personal Hygiene Feels Draining

Personal hygiene is one of those things that are crucial for your personal and social well-being. There is no doubt that keeping yourself clean, moisturized, and groomed leaves you feeling fresh and ready to tackle the day. This also makes it easy for people to interact with you. Overall, it's a positive thing, and most people enjoy having a good personal hygiene structure in their lives. However, it is not uncommon for some to find it challenging to do simple hygienic duties when they are experiencing a phase of poor emotional health. During such a time, showering, brushing your teeth, washing your hands, and doing laundry may start to feel like a difficult task to accomplish. The act or even just the thought of doing these things may bring about exhaustion and dread.

As a symptom of poor emotional health, people who feel drained by personal hygiene complain that they lack the stamina to perform routine self-care practices. This can be particularly complicated for black women who are mothers, as they not only have to tend to their own personal hygiene but also to their children's, which increases the negativity and exhaustion. Needless to say, feelings of guilt can easily join the party, creating a whirlwind of negative feelings and self-concepts.

The question that many of us ask is, why is it that something that was initially such a positive thing has now become so difficult and anxiety inducing? Researchers claim that exhaustion and a loss of interest in activities are two characteristics of serious, chronically poor emotional health. In other words, when you're emotionally unwell, you probably won't have much drive or energy to keep yourself clean.

It is not uncommon for people to describe their emotional exhaustion as a constant grey cloud or a feeling of being stuck beneath a pile of bricks. Poor emotional health feels like a heavy weight that makes it impossible for you to even want to get out of bed and go about the daily and often strenuous tasks of being a functional and thriving human being.

When you view emotional exhaustion through this lens, it becomes evident that the chores that people who are mentally healthy take for granted are enormous undertakings for those who are experiencing significant emotional exhaustion.

Emotional exhaustion does not just end in the realm of feelings, as it has a somatic side effect that is not only manifested in fatigue but in physical pain as well. Along with the abovementioned symptoms, black women experiencing poor emotional health will also experience negative bodily symptoms, which can make tending to their personal hygiene much harder.

Anxiety and Irritation

It is not uncommon for women who are experiencing poor emotional health to frequently feel extremely happy, extremely sad, or both. Their mood can fluctuate rather dramatically, making it difficult for them to live a stable and balanced lifestyle. A few mood disorders also include other enduring feelings like anger and irritation.

Generally, fluctuating moods based on the circumstances of life are a natural thing, and a person can only be diagnosed with mood disorder if the systems are present for a few weeks or more. Mood problems can alter behavior and make it difficult for people to carry out daily tasks, like working.

It's common for people to occasionally experience bouts of anxiety. Being anxious isn't always a bad thing. It may energize us, keep us vigilant, alert us to dangers, and inspire us to find solutions to our problems. However, if anxiety interferes with your capacity to function in daily life, it may be a problem. Anxiety can be an indication of a mental health issue if it is chronic, strong, difficult to regulate, or completely disproportionate to your current life circumstances.

Another symptom of emotional distress is irritability. Being irritable means you're more prone to get frustrated or upset quickly. It could happen in response to difficult circumstances. It could also be a sign of physical or mental health issues. Several factors can cause someone to become irritable. Physical and psychological factors can be used as broad categories to separate the reasons.

High Blood Pressure

There is a strong connection between poor emotional health and high blood pressure.

According to data from the American Heart Association, over 100 million persons in the US are considered to have hypertension, making high blood pressure a very common condition.

Your body's blood is continuously pumped by your heart, and as it does so, pressure is built up inside your arteries and against the walls of your blood vessels and veins. This pressure can increase dramatically, which leads to an excessively high movement force. Your blood vessels deteriorate over time if your blood pressure is kept high.

Most people are aware that having chronic hypertension raises your chance of having a heart attack or stroke. Still, you might not be aware that having uncontrolled or inadequately treated hypertension also jeopardizes your emotional health. Compared to people with normal blood pressure, those who have hypertension are more prone to suffer from mood disorders such as depression and anxiety.

Practical steps like having a diet filled with heart-healthy foods, exercising frequently, decreasing weight, and stopping smoking can make a big difference in how high blood pressure is managed. Medication is another option that can be exercised when making lifestyle modifications that aren't enough to manage your blood pressure.

Even just learning that you have hypertension can make people worried. But it's crucial to understand that with the right care, you can lower your blood pressure and safeguard your heart and emotional health. You're not doomed to die from a stroke or heart attack just because you have high blood pressure.

According to research on the link between high blood pressure and emotional health, it can have the following effects on your mental health:

Inflammation

Inflammation that is chronic and low-grade is brought on by hypertension. Your emotional health may suffer as a result of the chemicals associated with chronic inflammatory reactions interacting with the neurotransmitters that control your mood.

Increased Stress

The amount of stress-related substances circulating in your blood rises when hypertension is left untreated. Stress-related chemicals raise blood pressure, which leads to a vicious cycle. Your emotional health will suffer as a result of this reciprocal interaction.

Low Self-Esteem

There are definite connections between how we feel about ourselves and our general mental and emotional well-being, even while low self-esteem is not considered a mental health problem in and of itself. Self-esteem is described as the feelings and conceptions that a person has about themselves and the things that they do in life. Therefore, a person with a high level of self-esteem thinks of themselves as good, is able to identify their positive traits, and typically aspires to live a happy and successful life. A person with low self-esteem feels terrible about themselves and thinks they are unworthy of achievements, love, or pleasure.

This is a potentially hazardous way to live, as research has linked low self-esteem to emotional health problems and a poor quality of life. Listed below are just a few ways that having low self-esteem can impact your mental health and steps you can take to elevate it.

Relationship Problems

The relationships we cultivate with those who are closest to us help shape who we are as people because, as humans, we grow and learn about ourselves through our interactions with others. Negative feelings and a pessimistic view of oneself could result from bad relationships.

Addiction

According to psychological research, having low self-esteem as a child or young adult may increase one's risk of being addicted later in life. Alcohol and other drugs are frequently used by addicts to help them cope with their self-doubt. But over time, this form of escape turns into an addiction, which obviously has a negative impact on their pre-existing low levels of self-esteem.

Low self-esteem frequently coexists in a vicious cycle with other emotional health issues like emotional eating, high blood pressure, and anxiety. It's difficult to determine which happens first, but the combination is both frequent and problematic. The societal stigma surrounding emotional fragility may cause someone who already has issues maintaining their emotional health to experience a decline in self-esteem.

Building self-esteem is essential to become stronger in the face of all of life's difficulties. We learn to truly and honestly love ourselves despite all of our shortcomings and insufficiencies when we work toward a better life. This means pursuing healthier relationships, a more rewarding professional or occupational life, and abstinence from addiction. It can be extremely difficult to change our deeply ingrained feelings about ourselves, and experts frequently advise counseling to address the underlying causes of our self-deprecating beliefs.

The solution is to confront and transform these detrimental notions into more constructive ones.

It's also crucial to learn to cherish and take care of your body and mind by leading a healthy lifestyle. Regaining physical and mental confidence can start with a healthy diet, regular exercise, and meditation. It's crucial to really engage with the people we love and see the value of life and all its complexity. Most importantly, self-esteem can be greatly boosted when we feel loved and encouraged by those around us.

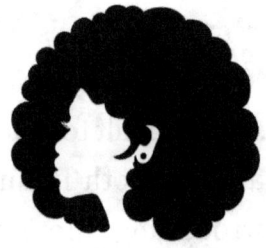

Chapter 4: How to Improve Your Emotional Health

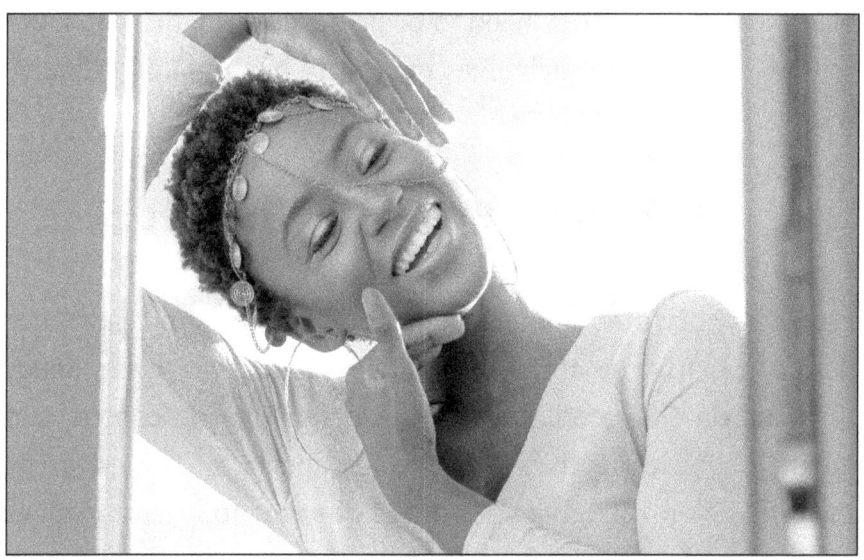

Being able to manage the totality of one's emotions and behavior is a sign of emotional wellness. Having solid emotional stability allows people to build good relationships and handle life's obstacles. The work required to maintain your emotional health is equal to or more than that needed to keep your physical health.

Never going through difficult times or having emotional issues doesn't imply that one is emotionally stable. Emotional hardships are common facets of life, and they can lead to anxiety, depression, and stress. The distinction is that resilient individuals possess good emotional health. This means that these individuals possess the necessary tools to deal with the vicissitudes of existence. They are able to maintain their composure and adaptability during difficult and trying times.

Learning how to improve your emotional health should be a priority as a black woman. Unfortunately, life isn't as kind to black women, and they need to be armored with an extra layer of tools to navigate their lives in a more healthy and effective way.

Nurture a Positive Mindset

Positively oriented beliefs, values, thoughts, and attitudes define a positive mentality. A positive mentality is the tendency to focus on the good things, expect positive outcomes, and tackle obstacles with a positive perspective. This strategy includes acknowledging your own skills and abilities as well as attempting to see the best in every situation and everyone. Even though it may sound cliche, having a positive outlook does not mean ignoring or avoiding difficult or unpleasant situations; rather, it means altering how you would approach such situations with the goal of achieving the most positive outcome.

Expecting to always be happy, only thinking positive thoughts, and being optimistic is highly unrealistic because those feelings aren't always justified. Life does get hard, and sometimes acknowledging the difficulty of a situation is healthier than faking positivity. But this is where each individual should learn how to practice a wise sense of distinction. Sometimes, being positive is exactly what you need to get you out of the gutter, and sometimes, not so much.

Positive thinking recognizes that having negative feelings is common. Unfortunately, we are not always able to control our thoughts or our emotions. Still, by accepting them, you may get past the unpleasant feelings and more easily decide how you will react to adversity. This acceptance of negative feelings tends to reduce their duration and severity. It's important to avoid becoming bogged down by bad feelings, as long-term negativity can lead to mental illnesses if they are left unchecked.

Positive thinkers are frequently more upbeat, thoughtful, and resilient. According to research, having a positive outlook is linked to better health, better stress management, a lower risk of heart disease, and lower rates of depression.

Thinking positively makes you speak and act more optimistically, which has a beneficial effect on your values, habit, and future. Although theoretically, this may sound extremely appealing, how exactly does one go about thinking more positively without tapping into the toxic positivity mindset?

When faced with problems in life, practicing positive thinking does not mean burying your head in the sand. It's not about ignorance or ignoring issues, as is frequently assumed. It means tackling challenging situations more productively and positively. Most importantly, it should be supported by logic and reason.

Positive thinking includes a number of perspectives on reality, namely:
- a positive outlook when tackling obstacles
- minimizing the effects of potentially negative circumstances
- attempting to see the best in others

- thinking positively about yourself and your abilities

Repetition is the bedrock of learning, and our psychological characteristics and conditions contribute significantly to our physical health. Unfortunately, the organ that we need the most, our heart, also suffers the most when we are under a lot of stress, frequently feel angry, or are nervous. People who showed optimism and a positive outlook had a much lower risk of cardiovascular disease. There are two plausible reasons for this, both of which are accurate. The first is that individuals with positive outlooks practice healthier habits, such as eating healthy foods, working out frequently, rarely smoking, and consuming less alcohol. Our crucial organ systems, particularly the cardiovascular system, are at risk from stress-related hormones and neurotransmitters.

It's okay to acknowledge that everyone experiences occasional anxiety or depression and that these feelings occasionally become intolerable to the point where we turn to medical assistance. Excessive worrying, which is a hallmark of generalized anxiety disorder, can be rewired to be replaced by positive thinking, according to research done on individuals who experienced it. Following a four-week course in positive imagery, the participants reported having fewer anxious thoughts.

Similar principles apply to treating depression: a cognitive-behavioral treatment approach advises changing negative beliefs with realistic and uplifting ones in order to lessen depressive symptoms. A positive mindset generally fosters mindfulness and happy feelings, which help our psychological health as a whole.

It functions similarly to how physical health does. All of this can be summed up by the idea of psychological capital. Resilience, hope, and optimism are three psychological resources that offer superior coping techniques. People with greater psychological capital are more devoted to and content with their professions. At work, they frequently do better and experience less pressure or anxiety. This is especially beneficial for black women, who tend to either work multiple jobs or stand as the sole breadwinner of the household. Positive thinking can create happier workers, and happier workers are more productive, creative, and get higher supervisor ratings. Consequentially, they earn more money as well. This demonstrates that encouraging a positive outlook has advantages for both individuals and the company. It is even safe to think that over time, you can actually increase your wealth by choosing to become a more positive, connected, and happier version of yourself.

Smile More

One of life's most simple yet most joyous things is smiles and laughter. Our smiles and laughter, though perceived as a relatively trivial aspect of most days, have greater effects on our emotional stability and well-being than we realize. Studies have shown a vast array of advantages of both, including improvements in our social lives, physical and mental health, and even longer lifespans.

True laughter spontaneously arises from a funny conversation or a happy moment. Having said that, we don't always laugh or smile when we're actually happy and content. Humans actually smile for a variety of reasons, such as to be polite or come off as accessible. In some cases, smiling is even done when we feel uncomfortable or scared, so it's an activity that can occur in vastly different situations but that ultimately seeks to serve the same purpose.

Researchers discovered that smiling activates two facial muscles. The first muscle is known as the zygomatic major, which regulates our mouth's corners. This muscle can be used whenever we desire. The second muscle, called the orbicularis oculi, regulates the region around our eyes. This muscle cannot be consciously activated. This implies that we only truly laugh or smile, what is now known as a Duchenne smile, when our eyes and mouth are open.

More recent studies have added to the evidence that smiles aren't always the result of pure joy or enjoyment. Smiling is a social cue focused on interaction rather than being motivated by an inner sense of joy. Participants in a study answered questions on a computer. It was discovered that participants smiled when they interacted with the computer, and interestingly, they smiled more frequently when they gave erroneous answers. This discovery was linked to a Darwinian method of behavior analysis called behavioral ecology theory, which studies the impact of evolution on human behavior.

A sincere smile, in the opinion of some academics, reflects the inner state of joy or amusement. However, according to behavioral ecology theory, being cheerful is neither required nor sufficient for the act of smiling. This theory asserts that all smiles are social interactional tools.

Numerous studies imply that we likely smile because it makes us feel happy and because it's necessary for our social interactions. Similar principles apply to laughter. There are two varieties of laughter: social and involuntary. The two most significant types of laughter, or distinctions between laughters, are whether or not it is entirely involuntary and whether or not it is a little more communicative.

Similar to smiling, laughter can arise spontaneously or as a result of social engagement. When you laugh uncontrollably, your body sometimes feels like it is being taken over by the laughter. Contrarily, social laughter is a controlled aspect of interactions. We laugh a lot to show that we know someone, that we like someone, and that we belong to the same group as someone. It is a social dance that says, "I see you and I am here with you."

There are numerous advantages of smiling and laughing for both our physical and mental health. People who smile more, whether on purpose or by default, live happier and longer lives. These are some of the advantages of bringing more smiles and laughter into your life.

You Become More Approachable

There are social advantages to smiling at other people. Perhaps you've heard that laughter spreads quickly. Studies support the validity of this. This brain response, which instinctively primes us to laugh or smile, offers a means for us to mimic other people's behavior, which is something that facilitates social interaction. Smiling and laughing could be crucial in creating solid ties between group members.

In other words, when you smile or laugh, it's likely that others will do the same, which will help you build relationships and spread happiness.

Your Body Discharges Positive Hormones

When you smile, your body releases three feel-good hormones, namely dopamine, endorphins, and serotonin. These let your body know that you are content, which makes you feel better. A single smile can stimulate the brain at a similar pace that 1,000 chocolate bars would. In fact, you'll feel better even if you fake a smile. Even while a forced smile might not be a Duchenne smile, doing so can actually improve your mood. It's interesting to note that a British study even claimed people who used Botox and were physically unable to frown felt happier overall.

You Forge Better Relationships

A smile is a universal language of love. Smiling and laughing foster friendship and aid in the formation of social relationships. Studies have shown a link between emotional well-being and laughter. In a 2015 study, psychologists videotaped 71 couples discussing their initial encounters. They discovered that relationship quality, intimacy, and social support were all positively correlated with how much of the talk involved mutual laughter. Laughter conveys that two people are a part of something together, as was previously stated. As a result, it deepens links and relationships.

Improved Work Productivity

Increased performance and productivity at work are directly connected with greater energy, faster promotions, better reviews, higher income, better health, and enhanced contentment with life. The employees who were happy were more productive. The happiest workers were 155% more content with their occupations and had 180% more energy. As a result, they spent 80% of their week on work-related activities compared to the 40% their unhappiest peers spent. Since a vast majority of us spend a significant portion of our lives at work, it's critical to feel content in order to feel successful. So, it's advantageous to start laughing and smiling more at work.

Stress Relief

There is ample evidence that laughing reduces stress. By lowering blood pressure and heart rate, laughter can calm down your stress reaction and make you feel more at ease. Additionally, laughter increases blood flow, which aids in muscular relaxation and over time lessens the physical signs of stress. You'll also receive a wide dose of dopamine, endorphins, and serotonin to improve your mood throughout the day. Even in trying situations, smiling and laughing can really make it easier to handle stress and overcome the situation with your sense of positivity still intact.

You Could Live Longer

Women with great senses of humor lived longer than other women, according to a 15-year Norwegian study that was published in April 2016. In fact, they had an 83% lower risk of contracting an infection and a 73% lower risk of dying from heart disease. Organs are stimulated by laughter. It can increase the amount of oxygen you take in, energize your heart and muscles, and lower your blood pressure and pulse rate. Black women may combat the physical impacts of aging by reducing stress, improving their social interactions, and feeling happier overall.

It's all good and well to want to start smiling and laughing more, but it can be difficult to get into this practice, especially if you are used to being a bit more on the gloomy side. Here are some strategies you may use to promote more smiles and laughter in your life:

- The first step to happiness is smiling even when you don't feel like it because even a phony smile can improve your sense of happiness.
- Watch a funny movie, read some jokes, or look for a humor boost in any method that makes you laugh if you're feeling sad or if you noticed that you haven't laughed in a while.
- Talk to people: We are conditioned to smile and laugh more in a group setting.
- Spend time with positive friends who encourage you.

- Don't take yourself too seriously; make fun of yourself. Your attitude is the key to success in life. Even when things are difficult, try to find the humor or the positive in the situation. Your attitude, your health, and your general quality of life will all benefit from this.

Seek and Accept Help and Support From Others

Everybody yearns to be the recipient of love and consideration from others. However, despite the fact that receiving may be advantageous to us and fulfill our desires for belonging and connection, it can also be an uncomfortable task for many of us. We have developed the unhealthy habit of thinking that less is better. Black women, in particular, have been known to carry the weight of the world on their shoulders while rarely asking for help or guidance from others. They may resist accepting things in general when they feel like a burden or an imposition on others. As a result, their contradictory reactions to receiving help can leave them more frustrated and isolated than before.

These nuanced responses to receiving may have some roots in our past experiences with attachment. Early attachments play a role in determining how we interact with others and the expectation we have of others interacting with us. We may feel less safe or trusting in the relationships we form as adults if we had an uneasy pattern of attachment as children.

It can be difficult or perplexing to accept this type of secure attachment-based help from others throughout our lives if we weren't accustomed to receiving constant, high-quality care from our parents or other attachment figures. Human beings are wired for familiarity, and the unfamiliar, even if it is beneficial, is evolutionarily contrived to be seen as a threat.

Black women can find it challenging to rely on others for assistance. First of all, admitting they can't accomplish everything on their own can be difficult. When they admit that they truly need something from someone else, they may experience feelings of guilt and unresolved childhood traumas. This is particularly true if they experienced a difficult time having their needs met during the first year of their lives. These are the fundamentals of the avoidant attachment style, where the child learns to be independent and conceal their wants in order to prevent the excruciating feelings of shame that come from having their needs unmet. They can be concerned that expressing a need will be viewed as "too much" if they do.

When we have an avoidant attachment style, we often feel pseudo-independent and driven to take care of our own needs. This can make it more difficult to rely on or look for help from others. It could be difficult to imagine that things could turn out better than they did for us in the past. Allowing people to assist us or offer us anything can go against our belief that we should take care of our needs alone or not have any at all.

Asking for help or accepting help would require us to give up an adaptation that felt vital for survival when we were helpless, dependent children. Leaving behind something that made us feel safe can initially make us feel uneasy, uncertain, and even scared. These emotions will eventually pass as we become accustomed to a newfound and healthier reality in which we can embrace and take part in the giving and receiving with others and the intimacy it fosters.

Additionally, if we stated a need, we would have to let go of an early-on negative persona we created that viewed us as burdens or needy. Because a young child has to perceive their parent in the positive in order to feel protected, this identity develops. The child automatically assumes that it is their fault if a parent is not sensitive to or responsive to their needs, maintaining their perception of them as good parents.

As with any other skill, we can improve our ability to receive if we give it value. We must remove the internal walls that separate us from other people in order to do this. We can start by focusing on the "critical inner voices" that feed our apprehension and resistance to accepting help and ultimately accepting love. We might make an effort to be conscious of the unfavorable thoughts that surface when we receive recognition or compassion from others.

We might begin to investigate our attachment styles and how they might affect our capacity to receive generosity from others, in addition to disregarding and overtly acting against the counsel of our inner critic. Our affiliations may be the source of our sentiments of mistrust, unease, and feigned independence since they might serve as examples of how we anticipate other people will behave. Having a deep understanding of our attachment style might help us develop greater inner security and make us more welcoming of others.

We must shift our perspective from one of self-preservation to one of healthy interaction with people and strengthen our bonds with others if we are to become more adept at accepting help. When we accept more from others, we are able to offer more to others. That is the reciprocal relationship of the social animal. By denying ourselves, we also betray those who are dear to us. Everyone gains from generosity since it is a two-way street. We can never truly give with a genuinely open heart unless we can also receive with it. We either deliberately or unknowingly attach a sense of judgment to helping others when we do the same with receiving it. Happiness depends on our ability to give, but generosity also involves pushing ourselves to be gracious in our acceptance of that which others give us.

When we accept kindness from one another, both parties feel closer to each other. Rather than excluding them, we allowed them to express their love for us. This strengthens our bond with them and builds a stronger system of mutual support, where giving and receiving can feel organic and equitable. Despite any initial unease, accepting aid from others can be gratifying. Being vulnerable enough to embrace kindness and compassion tends to elicit positive reactions from other people and frequently results in closer emotional bonds.

Gratitude

Gratitude is the act of expressing gratitude for one's tangible or intangible valuables in life. It is an acknowledgment of the inherent value embedded in all things. It is an internal, spontaneous declaration of warmth and goodness. Relationships are strengthened by this social emotion, which has profound evolutionary foundations stemming from the survival necessity of assisting others and receiving support in return. According to studies, feeling and expressing thankfulness involves particular brain regions. When given a task that encourages the expression of appreciation, people's brain scans reveal long-lasting modifications in the prefrontal cortex that increase sensitivity to subsequent instances of gratitude. Focusing on gratitude is one of the most effective methods to reprogram your brain for more joy and less stress. Here are a few easy ways to express more gratitude in your life.

Start a Gratitude Journal

Make it a habit to remind yourself each day of the blessings, grace, advantages, and positive aspects you experience. You have the chance to weave a lasting theme of thankfulness into your life by reflecting on moments of gratitude connected to the everyday experiences of your life, your unique qualities, or important people in your life.

Reflect on the Negative

Remembering your past struggles can help you be appreciative of where you are right now. When you reflect on how challenging life was in the past and how far you have come, you establish an explicit understanding of where you currently are in your life. This contrast is a good place to start cultivating gratitude.

Express Your Gratitude to Others

Relationships can be strengthened by expressing your gratitude. Therefore, be sure to express your appreciation to your partner, friend, or family member the next time they accomplish something you value. This not only fortifies your existing relationships but makes you feel good in the process.

Get Your Act Together

Our five senses, touch, sight, smell, taste, and hearing, help us understand what it is to be a person and how miraculous it is to be alive. The human body is not just a miraculous creation; it is also a gift. This vessel carries you through life and fights off illnesses to keep you alive. If you are able-bodied, think of all the ways you can use your body daily.

Make a Commitment to Cultivate Gratitude

According to research, making a deep commitment to carry out a particular activity increases the likelihood that it will actually be done. Writing a gratitude pledge and even starting a daily gratitude journal practice can help you stay committed to finding the value and beauty in the day.

Watch What You Say

People who are grateful have distinctive language usage. They tend to use words like abundance, blessings, and fortune. Aside from this, they focus on the good things others do for them.

Chapter 5: The Race War

Black women have struggled with dual discrimination: they are black and women. This places them at the lower end of the social hierarchy in relation to other demographics. Black women haven't been able to enjoy the protection of their men and society, and the conflicting ideas of having to sacrifice their femininity in order to survive have made it extremely difficult for black women to generate a unified sense of identity that is not in constant conflict with itself. When we speak about the racial war, we see the image of the raped, abandoned, and disenfranchised black woman. Despite all of these odds, the black woman has fought ferociously to become something of value, not just in society but in herself.

From Then Till Today

Black women have traditionally fought on several fronts, such as those for civil rights, suffrage, the abolition of slavery, and eliminating segregation. Fighting has since become synonymous with the black woman's identity.

Black women have been fighting slavery even while it was legal. They fought back in Africa and in their communities. When they were violently captured and placed on ships, they fought back. When they were transported like sacks of potatoes on the Middle Passage, they fought back. These were women who, at the time, were considered to be African captives. The current generation of black women is not the first.

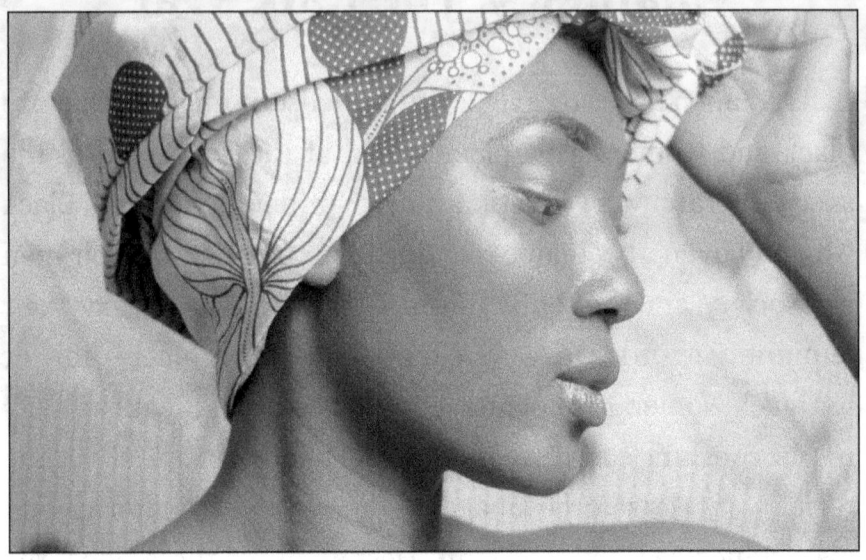

But it is also critical that we understand and acknowledge the fact that black women were not enslaved but immigrated to the United States. They faced and are still facing struggles. Although slavery in America was more overt, with shackles, chains, and violent midnight rapes by their slave masters, black women in Africa were slaves to their patriarchal systems. These are women who would be married off to a wealthy man in the village as soon as they bled for the very first time.

They joined a coalition of sister wives and were expected to breed and remain loyal to their husbands until their value expired and until he decided to marry a younger, more attractive female. Black women's agency hasn't been much of a reality for a very long time, so it's no wonder that their lives have been defined by a constant fight to prove themselves to the world.

There is a lot that is known about black women throughout the time of slavery, and this is because research in this area has advanced significantly since the 1980s. What is known is that black women throughout slavery did precisely what they believed was worth it: they fought for freedom, demanded justice, demanded to have their voices heard, fought to protect their bodies, and fought to protect their families.

Early regulation, dating back to the 1660s, stated that if black women had children, their children would likewise be sold into slavery if their mothers were slaves. According to a legislation known as *partus sequitur ventrem*, a Latin term that essentially means "of the belly," a person's status as an enslaved person was thus determined by their mother. Consequently, if your mother was a black slave, you were also a slave as soon as you were born. This resulted in a hereditary state of the institutionalization of slavery based on motherhood in the United States, thus, the wombs and uteruses of black women were now being traded for goods, and the same was true of their children and offspring. Black women quite literally were reduced into a commodity. Not very different from the black women who stayed on African soil, who were made to give birth to especially male children to continue the legacy and the bloodline of their male counterparts.

You may be reading this and thinking, "How exactly did they fight this?" When we consider what that means in early history, before the United States became the United States, when we consider how the systemic evolution of slavery is nestled on the wombs and bodies of black women, it does not imply that black women, as previously mentioned, were not resisting. Black women were indeed fighting at this time by using petitions for freedom. An example of a black woman fighting is Elizabeth Key. She went to court and presented her case with witnesses to attest that she too could or ought to be free, filed petitions, and also gathered supporters. She found success through this fight.

Black women were also battling for their freedom to speak out and defend their children. Sojourner Truth went before a grand jury to plead for her son's return, which was extraordinary for a black woman to do. According to some evidence, they initially mocked her, but she persisted and raised money to eventually, two years later, got back her son, who had been sold into slavery in the deep South.

When we consider the legacy that individuals like Stacey Abrams and Vice President Kamala Harris fall under, one of the things that we discover in the history of black women is that they are developing their own institutions. Black women have a long history of engaging in this kind of activism. We have women who were involved in slavery now participating in the women's suffrage movement because they were aware that black men received the vote before all women. In addition to this, although the 14th and 15th Amendments purported to provide universal citizenship, some African-American women were left out of that equation.

As a result of their systematic exclusion, black women seek out independent means of protest and strategies to create their own institutions and organizations. The National Organization of Colored Women, a group of colored women's clubs, was one of the organizations and was established in 1896.

These black women were organizing these clubs all around the country, and they weren't just concentrating on one issue. They frequently worked on several fronts. They worked on suffrage, antislavery, and the right to care for and raise their children as non-slaves. This had led black women to take an empowering and leading role in their lives. They were known to be strong and relentless, which eventually evolved into the notion of the empowering but equally perilous strong black woman trope. Black women are currently working with their entire body and soul, and often twice as hard as their male and white counterparts, to achieve half of what they get simply because they are still viewed as less than by society. And so, black women step further and further into the strong black women role, enduring hardships and difficulties, wearing themselves thin, and corroding themselves from within. This has led to a series of social misconceptions about that black woman that further alienates and places her in a perpetual vicious cycle.

Social Misconceptions

Black women have suffered from unfavorable stereotypes in mainstream American society as a result of slavery and its economic, social, and political repercussions. One of these stereotypes is the infamous trope of the angry black woman, which depicts these women as irrational, domineering, and antagonistic without cause. Black women's symptoms following mental health therapy may support this misconception.

Many of the angry black woman's unfavorable traits, however, were the result of environmental stressors and historical circumstances. Additionally, black women's expressions of rage impact how the mental health professional interprets the presenting symptoms.

This myth and associated unfavorable stereotypes have a major intrapsychic and interpersonal impact on black women, and they may also have an impact on how well mental health treatments work. Understanding the mythology of the angry black woman, including its origins, expressions, and the particular experiences of black women, may raise the bar for clinicians' cultural competence and lead to better therapeutic outcomes when dealing with this demographic.

Many facets of American culture, especially the workplace, have been affected by the trope of the angry black woman. This widespread misconception not only paints black women as being more hostile, confrontational, domineering, irrational, ill-tempered, and bitter, but it also may be keeping them from reaching their full potential in their professions and influencing their entire work experiences. Black women make up over 7% of the workforce, yet they are still underrepresented in leadership roles, with no black female CEOs in the Fortune 500. Researchers have looked into potential obstacles preventing black women from moving up the corporate ladder, such as limited access to social networking and fewer mentoring opportunities, in an effort to better understand the causes of underrepresentation.

People also have a tendency to ascribe black women's anger to internal causes, which is likely to have a detrimental impact on assessments of their work performance and leadership potential. Given that anger is a feeling that is frequently experienced and expressed at work, the stereotype of the angry black woman may have a detrimental effect on black women's job status and career advancement. It's important to highlight the trope as one of many elements that can have a damaging effect on a black woman's career. Understanding the obstacles that black women encounter in the workplace is a difficult problem.

This trope is even evident before black women enter the workforce. For instance, black female students at a university with a majority of white students reported experiencing microaggressions or snarky comments from other students and were aware of the stereotype of the irate black woman. Even if the message in a debate about college scholarships was the same, university students evaluated black female speakers as being angrier and ruder than white female speakers. Participants could choose 5 out of 92 characteristics that best described either black women or white women. Compared to white women, who were more likely to be described by characteristics like sensitivity, independence, and family values, black women were more likely to be described by characteristics like loud and strong.

Many black women have to watch their body language and facial expressions to make sure they appear calm and rational, calibrating themselves into a specific tone so as to not frighten or upset people in authority.

This makes them feel disingenuous. It interferes with their well-being and sense of worth. The angry black woman caricature constantly pressures women to act friendly in order to maintain a semblance of safety and likeability in a world that doesn't particularly like or protect black people.

Living in a society that affixes a dehumanizing stereotype to women who show typical human emotions has measurable repercussions. Black women are forced to hide their anger instead of expressing it, which causes it to fester and ache. Suppressed anger frequently contributes to mental health issues like depression, anxiety, and increased stress levels. Additionally, compared to white women, black women have more persistent and severe symptoms of anxiety. Black women are less likely to seek therapy for anxiety and depression and are more likely to receive harmful and inefficient care when they do.

Additionally, there is a physical aspect to this: The physical health problems that black women experience more frequently than white women, such as high blood pressure, heart disease, breast cancer, and diabetes-related death rates, are all caused by the excessive load black women carry, which includes repressed anger. None of these conditions are suitable for anxiety and depression.

Yes, black women have plenty of reasons to be outraged. No matter how hard they strive, anti-black bias and structural racism prevent them from often having the same fair chance as their white and non-black counterparts.

Black women are less successful on dating apps, less likely to marry and enjoy the physical, financial, and spiritual benefits that frequently accompany long-term partnerships, and less likely to be prescribed painkillers when they visit the doctor. They are more likely to die during childbirth; earn less; accumulate less wealth; are overrepresented in prisons and underrepresented in the corporate world; are less likely to be invited for interviews if they have stereotypical black names, more likely to be stopped by the police, and the list goes on. None of this is the result of an inherent lack of talent or focus on the part of black women. Mainstream society doesn't care about them as much as it does about others, despite the fact that they have made significant contributions to science, politics, art, law, philosophy, athletics, spirituality, music, and the very creation of the American nation.

Now, with your eyes closed, visualize a real, angry black woman, not a stereotype. Can you view her without the distorted, cartoonish perspective you have in mind? She is probably in agony and crying. She might be a mother, and her angry nature is really just the tenacity and fortitude that characterizes that position. She might be your supervisor, and her apparent rage is really just an honest reaction to how you performed. She might have only recently experienced a racial situation, or she might not be angry at all.

Real black women who are angry are complex, not flat, and can't be summed up by a stereotype. You are not a caricature. You are a complex, cultured, and intelligent human being. You have the right to experience and express the full range of human emotions. You are deserving of respect.

In certain cultures, black female anger is viewed as beautiful. Beautiful as a reaction against racism, misogyny, and injustice everywhere. Beautiful as an act of creation and resistance. Resistance against systemic, anti-black, and anti-woman racism.

The Effects of Racism on the Black Woman's Psyche

Black women are just as likely as other women to struggle with emotional wellness, but they are more likely to receive subpar or no treatment. Black women are frequently underrepresented in scientific research and reluctant to seek mental health treatment. This is due to various factors, including racism, the stigma associated with mental illness, and the past use of information by providers against patients. Additionally, it could be difficult for them to locate black or culturally appropriate therapists. Because of the myth that the strong black women can handle anything, certain clinicians who may not be culturally competent may also subscribe to it, further alienating women from the help that they need. That undermines a person's perspective, shows no empathy for what they are going through, and may even downplay their symptoms.

Misogynoir is a particular form of prejudice against black women that takes both race and gender into account. It is both racialized sexism and gendered racism. Evidence-based statistics on misogyny's effects on mental health are still lacking.

However, by examining the consequences racist and sexist encounters have on a person's mental well-being, a clear picture may be built. According to a study, one in five women reports experiencing sex-based discrimination. These women are more likely to experience severe emotional distress as a result of these encounters. The experiences of racial discrimination, according to many people of color, have left them feeling physically and psychologically uncomfortable as well as culturally and socially alienated.

Compared to women of other races, black women face higher stress levels, with racial issues being the main cause of such sentiments. Black women are more prone to experience chronic health issues such as high rates of hypertension, diabetes, obesity, lupus, maternal morbidity, and preterm birth due to these persistent pressures. The combination of these things traumatizes the mind and body.

For Black women, all racist experiences—medical, interpersonal, or institutional—combine to create an existence that is frequently and incessantly stressful. According to studies, this toxic stress encourages the body's inflammatory response at the cellular level. This inflammation is what causes preeclampsia, hypertension, dementia, and other chronic illnesses that black women are more likely to develop or die from. Black people are more likely than Hispanic or white people to suffer premature death, that is, dying before they reach the age of 75. The health disparities are shocking, and racism-induced stress has unavoidable negative repercussions on mental health.

Naturally, gender bias affects how women are treated and how their pain is managed, but black women also experience racial bias in addition to the former. According to studies, doctors and medical students assume black people can tolerate more pain than non-black folks. Myths about black people's thicker skin and reduced pain threshold contribute to poor pain management, with black women who report pain to medical practitioners typically receiving 22% fewer prescriptions for painkillers.

Not only are these encounters traumatic, but they are frequently lethal. Breast cancer is one incredible example of this deeply embedded racial inequality. Black women are more likely to die from breast cancer but are less likely to get diagnosed. Black women die from breast cancer at a rate that is 40% greater than that of white women. Doctors are more likely to diagnose breast cancer in its earliest stages in white women than in black women.

Systemic racism is the cause of the many racial health disparities that exist. Racism was a foundational principle of America. It shouldn't come as a surprise that the practice of medicine is also rife with racism because the practice of medicine was founded on racism. Racism continues to cause black women to have unequal access to employment opportunities, which leads to unequal access to adequate medical care and insurance. It is crucial to pay attention to and take care of black women's health since gender bias and racism have a negative impact on both mental and physical well-being.

Chapter 6: Find Confidence in Your Blackness

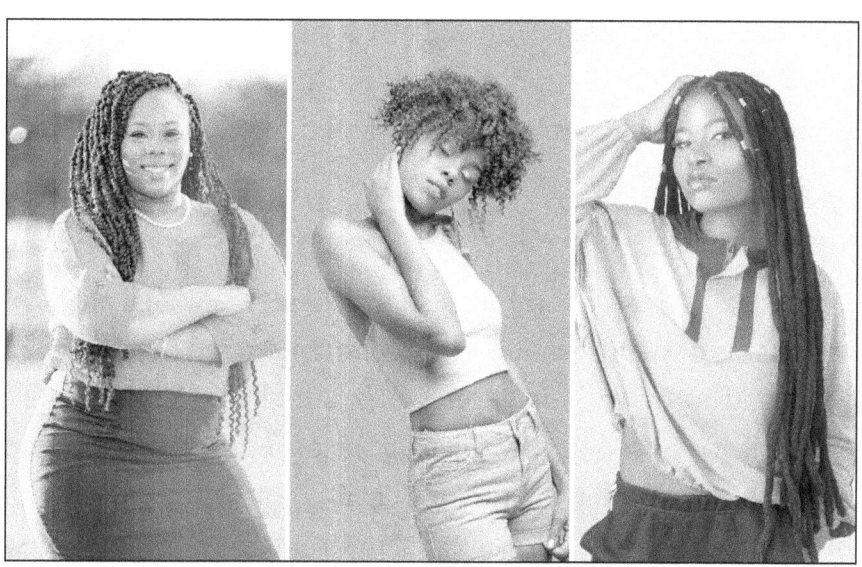

Self-love is accepting that you are not able to achieve everything. You don't have superpowers. You definitely have some skills and unique qualities, but you also have some weaknesses, and it's crucial that you learn how to accept them. Black women have several qualities, and they are undeniably beautiful. The most important thing that a black woman can learn to do is accept herself for who she is, flaws and all. Arm yourself in all your beauty and pain. Find confidence in the truth of all that you are.

The Physical

Black women's bodies have been vandalized, scrutinized, and villainized for centuries. This ranges from brutal slave rapes to the over-sexualization and objectification of black women's bodies in mainstream media. It is hard to say if black women have ever felt truly in charge of their own bodies. There are two prominent features that stand out when we discuss black women's bodies, namely their hair and their curves.

Hair

Wigs and extensions are mostly purchased by black women, and in this day and age, it is quite common to find black women who tend to wear their natural hair under these Eurocentric and Asiatic caps. Some of this is done as a protection method due to the inherent brittle and easily damageable nature of black women's hair. However, some women do this because they are fundamentally uncomfortable with their natural hair. Black women have been made to feel inferior when it comes to their hair since slavery. The tighter curls were not celebrated, and relaxers were introduced as a way to tame the afros on their heads. This led to centuries of self-hate. The term "good hair" arose as praise to black women—usually biracial women with looser curl patterns—having hair that was more socially acceptable and manageable.

Black women have greater anxiety related to their hair and are twice as likely as white women to experience pressure at work to straighten it. A significant portion of people displays implicit racial bias against black women's hair texture.

Black women have endured discrimination for their skin tone, physical characteristics, and unprocessed hair for as long as they have lived in America.

African hair was thought to be more similar to sheep wool than human hair by British colonists in the 18th century, setting the standard of white hair being better or "good," which is in and of itself a racially charged idea. Many African Americans tried to relax their hair to fit in after slavery was abolished. The first black woman to become a millionaire, Madame C.J. Walker, got rich by selling goods designed to relax black hair so that black women may advance in society by looking like the majority.

Conversely, there was a counter-movement, particularly nestled in the liberation movement, that sought to reclaim the natural hair of black women as a sense of power and an identifying factor of blackness. The 1960s saw a rise in the popularity of protest haircuts due to a desire for revolution and an expression of black pride. The Afro was the best illustration of this concept. The Afro was not only regarded as a political statement, but it was also well-liked by the media.

When black youth started wearing the Afro, activists, performers, and other people started noticing it. Celebrities like Diana Ross and The Jackson 5 became avid wearers of the afro hairdo.

Since then, the significance of African-American hair has grown within black communities. Black hair is crucial to black women's identity. Although black women with straight hair have more employment opportunities and social prospects both within and outside the black community, the diminished sense of self that is felt by adopting Eurocentric ideals of beauty has given rise to a group of black women who opt to wear their hair naturally.

It appears that black women are choosing to embrace their natural hair to the fullest extent possible as the natural beauty movement spreads across the US. According to a recent study, black women are more inclined to style their hair naturally without using any chemicals or heat. 51% of black women claim that their current hairstyle gives them a confidence boost and helps them feel beautiful.

Most black women believe that healthy hair equates to beautiful hair, and the black haircare market has adjusted to the new standard of natural hair. As more women feel emboldened to adopt an Afrocentric beauty look, a growing number of them are making the deliberate decision to wear their natural hair. Black women should be encouraged to unashamedly embrace their styled, natural selves through brands with a product designed exclusively for natural hair. When possible, black women can also opt to use natural ingredients to be healthy on the inside. This can also be reflected in the products and tools they use to maintain and style their hair.

Curves

Black women's bodies were vandalized and commodified during slavery. To put the cherry on top, black bodies were not seen as the standard of beauty, as black women tend to be curvier on average than non-black women. This has undoubtedly affected the confidence levels of black women, but there has been a significant shift in recent years.

A pattern emerged in survey after survey. Black women consistently reported having higher self-esteem than Hispanic or white women, and among other things, they were significantly more likely to describe themselves as successful and beautiful. These studies show that race affects self-confidence. Given the lengthy history of prejudice and discrimination they have experienced, it may seem surprising that research indicates black women have higher self-esteem than women of other races and ethnicities.

When black women look in the mirror, they also have more positive thoughts about themselves and their bodies. This new generation of black women is taught as they grow up that they are intelligent, strong, and beautiful by their families. This mentality is passed down from one generation to the next as a defensive mechanism against racial discrimination. Black women believe that arming themselves with an unwavering sense of confidence and love for their bodies will allow them to become better able to handle racism.

That might also help to explain why black women embraced their curvy bodies long before it was trendy to do so in the mainstream media. Curvy bodies were always praised in black culture, even though the Eurocentric model celebrated otherwise. Black women claim that this internal assurance can be a potent remedy for a culture that occasionally feels unfriendly and unwelcoming to black bodies.

Black women can begin their journey towards building physical confidence by embracing the very things that have been rejected and demonized by society.

You should look at the parts of you that you find unattractive and honestly examine whether it is genuinely something that you believe or a notion that has been instilled in you. Whether you are curvy, skinny, light-skinned, dark-skinned, tall, short, biracial, or unambiguously black, you are beautiful and deserving to be here.

The Emotional

Society applauds the strong black woman trope, with its essence of invincible superhuman strength, as verbal credentials and congratulatory ideals of strength and appreciation to the collective perseverance of black women. However, this racist trope rooted in white supremacist society has been able to keep black women trapped in a detrimental narrative for centuries. It praises the black woman for how well she manages to keep her complex issues and dynamic emotions from being expressed and affecting the lives of others while also tearing her down, utilizing her labor, and working tirelessly to diminish her worth.

Black women are caught in a trap that dehumanizes and renders them defenseless. The strong black woman trope is nestled in the colonial shackles that draw its inspiration from the "mammy" image and capitalizes on the perception of a lack of women as strong, independent individuals who don't need anyone's help because "she's got this!"

This trope benefits from the ancestral resilience of black women. She is a single mother who manages her home while working multiple jobs.

She struggles while receiving welfare but yet somehow finds a way to make ends meet for her children. Either that or she is a highly educated workaholic with a dismal love life who is unlikely to get married and is so difficult to love that not even black men are willing to propose to her. Perhaps it doesn't matter what she does or how she chooses to live her life because the black woman's existence in a colonial environment has been built in such a way that she is a natural stress endurer, even if she does not have a fantastic love and sex life.

Dealing with stress, emotional conflict, and ongoing dependence on others seems normal due to the systematic psychological violation that permeates black women's communities, homes, and lives. From a very young age, black women learn routines for emotional restraint or numbness, along with a continual supply of self-reliance and tenacity. The strong black women trope means that black women's needs always come after. She is expected to take care of everyone around her first, and often, her own emotional needs become an afterthought or not even a thought at all.

She is also expected to have no expectations in return. She must provide for herself because she is responsible for herself. She never complains, and she never gets worn out by the difficulties life may present. She does not cry. She does not complain. And if she does, it is behind closed doors, in the silence of her pain and suffering. And the world applauds her for it. The world wants her to continue to be it. The world "loves" the black woman, so as long as she can continue to be a strong black woman. Ultimately, this trope is so insidious that it renders her emotionally incapacitated and crippled.

When a black woman displays symptoms of stress and emotion, this portrays her as being weak, dependent, or attention-seeking. It is thought that seeking validation from others is an indication of low self-esteem. The black woman has been brainwashed to be seen as a more capable trauma survivor and faster healer than other women. This conditioning actually served as a justification for white people's violence against black women when the strong black woman trope was established during slavery. The notion that black female slaves were strong enough to endure any pain and carry on justified slaveowners' abuses, including rape, solidified the black woman's mythic "strength" and became a potent justification for every violation committed against her.

The Jezebel caricature gave origin to the mythical "strength" that is used to justify the horrific abuses done to black women, helping to destroy their humanity as a result of the process of hyper-sexualization. The black woman's mental health and emotional well-being, which are inextricably linked to her humanity, were erased as a direct result of this dehumanization.

Promoting the stereotype of the strong black woman is problematic and unrealistic. If you heavily subscribe to this notion, you fall prey to unknowingly depriving yourself of the chance to be open and vulnerable, to address your most fundamental needs, and to take care of yourself by internalizing it. It supports the false notion that putting yourself first is superfluous at best and self-serving at worst, regardless of whether you're still helping others around you.

The strong black woman stereotype is exhausting, and you should seek to maintain a mindset and habits that support you, validate your value to others, and maintain your physical, mental, and emotional health. You should stop being an afterthought. You are deeply important and valuable.

There are so many common misconceptions about self-care. Even more adversely, black women are impacted by these beliefs. Self-care is not a sign of weakness or selfishness. Self-care is a survival tactic. So, let's redefine strong black women to include self-care.

Let us take the example of Simone Biles, who, at 24 years old and at the peak of her gymnastic career, opted to withdraw from several Olympic events to prioritize rest and her mental health. The world went absolutely crazy when they heard this, and several news reporters and commentators called her selfish and lazy. But black women, strong black women, should know that she was not any of those things at that moment. Simone Biles is a gymnast. Her strength is visible in her lithe and muscular body. Her strength is present in her work ethic, with years of training and discipline to become one of the best Olympians of her time. Her strength is in her ability to outperform her peers and stand proudly as a beautiful and successful black woman. And most importantly, her strength is in her ability to know how to give herself grace and rest when she most needs it. Self-care, true self-care for emotional wellness, is about knowing when to pull the plug. Black women have been overworked and over-independent for centuries. It's beautiful that we are able to fight so ferociously for the things that we want.

It is amazing that we are able to be so resilient in the face of adversity. And it should also be celebrated when we acknowledge that we are tired, we need a break, and we need to rest.

Your ability to give yourself room to feel, like any other human does, will imbue you with a sense of confidence and self-love that is difficult to shake. Knowing that you are doing something to take care of yourself—even if the world doesn't agree—is the most powerful act of self-love and self-care. Your emotional well-being matters, my dear black woman. You deserve to cry, to express your exhaustion, and to rest. You deserve to be taken care of as well. You deserve to live. Start choosing yourself and your well-being.

Stepping away from the Olympic stage, even for a moment, helped Simone Biles realize she was so much more than her gymnastics record. Black women everywhere should also understand that they are more than their accomplishments. Keep in mind that you don't need to be a professional athlete or a celebrity to deserve time off, to be kind to yourself, to step back and give your mental health and well-being some attention, or to deserve relaxation. I beg you, black women, take a break. Don't just make your mental health a priority; protect it passionately and with reckless abandon because no one else will.

The Spiritual

According to a number of studies, religion is crucial for the mental health and happiness of black women and helps them deal with social and personal challenges. A recent study suggests that spirituality, not religion, maybe the factor most crucial to the psychological health of black women.

Even though they are related, earlier research has demonstrated that black women see religion and spirituality as two different things. The participation of an individual in religious practices and commitment to predetermined beliefs are frequently used to describe religiousness. On the other side, spirituality involves relational and meaning-making aspects, such as forging a relationship with a higher power and feeling a connection to other people and the universe.

Adhering to religious ideology or participating in religious activities may not be as important to black women's life satisfaction and mental health as how they understand the meaning of their relationships.

In a study conducted online of over 160 black women, religious and spiritual beliefs and practices were examined. The participants ranged from ages 20 to 75. More than 60% of individuals, who identified as middle class, had graduate or professional degrees. The participants' psychological health, general life satisfaction, and level of religiosity, as demonstrated by their engagement in religious practices and adherence to shared religious values, were all evaluated. Their spirituality, including their link with a higher force or universal intelligence, their views on nature, and their sense of purpose in life, were also evaluated. 79% of the black women reported being roughly to highly spiritual, while less than 1% of respondents claimed to be not spiritual at all.

The study indicated that black women with higher levels of spirituality experienced a better mental health profile. They were happier with their lives, and that spirituality fully moderated the links between religiosity, mental health, and life satisfaction.

Spirituality's full mediation of the association between religiosity and life happiness suggests that participants' ties to others and supernatural beings, coupled with meaning-making practices, maybe the reason for this heightened sense of well-being. According to the results of the study, spirituality rather than religiosity may directly account for black women's high psychological well-being.

Now, this isn't so much about black women not adhering specifically to religious institutions like Christianity or Islam, but more so about them finding a deep sense of meaning in that. And spirituality, which is more about the connection of the spirit with the divine, be it God or some supernatural force, is what brings about this profound sense of belonging and connectedness. In that process, black women find that their confidence increases. Enslaved black women of the past found ways to merge their ancestral religious beliefs with Christianity. Examples of these are the Brazilian women who practice Candomblé and worship deities of the Yoruba religion in Nigeria while simultaneously fusing some Catholicism into their practice. These women have found a way to feel confident in their blackness by merging the roots of their spiritual past with their spiritual present.

Ultimately, it is about finding a deep sense of connection to something divine. If fusing ancestral elements into your spiritual practice helps you find more confidence in your blackness, then do it. You want to reach a point where you feel comfortable expressing yourself however you feel is best for you, and being true to yourself is the only way that you can reach that point. Spirituality is an incredibly personal and intimate part of our lives. Black women should not have to feel like the way in which they connect to the divine is another form of conformity and oppression. Black women should find their own sense of truth and pursue that with all their hearts. At the end of the day, when all is said and done, it is just you and God.

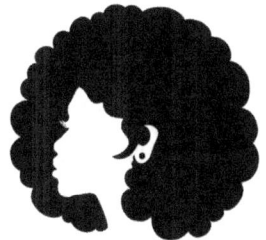

Chapter 7: Prepare for the Road Ahead

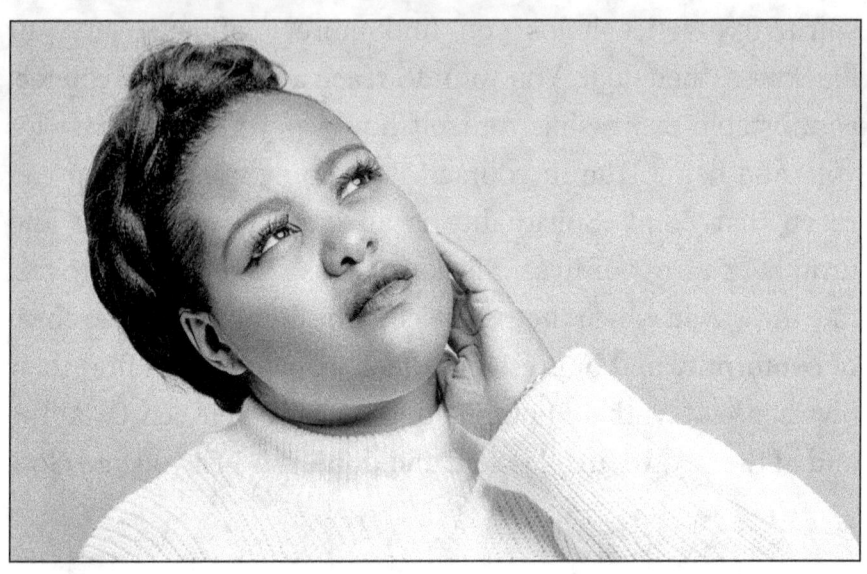

Learning how to un-learn the problematic and limiting ideals perpetuated by society for several centuries can be a project of a lifetime. Even if you do manage to transform your psyche and perceive things from a different lens, the world may not be on par with the speediness of your transformation process, making it even more complicated to coincide with your inner and outer reality. This is where a proposed modification of the strong black woman trope can be re-introduced. You need to learn how to be strong enough to fight the voices in your head that say you are not good enough. You need to start small, and value every bit of incremental progress you make, and not think of yourself as a failure if you relapse into old thought processes and behaviors. You need to understand being a black woman is a tiny percentage of who you are.

Love Yourself More

Black women's dehumanization has a long and complicated history. Many people have been trained not to view black women as entirely human, credible, or desirable, especially those with dark skin. In certain instances, society has been trained not to even notice black women. You were taught as a child that being lighter was better. It is not uncommon for black women to report the startling experiences they had as children when other lighter or white children bullied them or asked why they were the same color as "poo-poo." These experiences completely tarnished the self-concept of black women, who at a young age are already taught that a women's value is in her beauty, only to be radically rejected by society at such a young and fragile age. Those are the effects of being compared to feces by classmates who won't play with them on the playground, leading to little girls as young as four trying to wash their skin off. The imagery is harrowing in and of itself. Seeing a young and defenseless child trying to desperately change the unchangeable and realizing that they are stuck in a body that the entire world rejects. How can a little girl develop self-esteem and a positive self-concept in this way? How can she feel valuable if the world denies her like this from the very moment she is born? How can she love herself?

To have the boldness to love oneself as a black woman is a revolutionary act given this daily exposure to these, at best, boring and, at worst, terrifying circumstances.

Self-love has many faces, but at the heart of the unconditional acceptance that is the bedrock of true love, accepting your limitations is a key component of self-love. You have to acknowledge that you are all too human and do not have superpowers. You most certainly have some skills and special qualities, but you also have some weaknesses, and you should learn how to accept them. You are flawed, and that makes you human. I begin by stating the acceptance of one's flaws because therein lies the true fight. It is easy to see the parts of yourself that make you desirable and attractive and latch on to them as a lifeboat while you sail the rocky shores of your turbulent existence. But accepting your flaws means letting go of that lifeboat and becoming one with the treacherous waters. Predicting their unpredictability and ultimately finding a sense of order in the chaos. This is not only the act of loving oneself but the act of living in and of itself, and so, facing your flaws and your deepest fears is what makes you indeed come alive. There is a deep power that is harnessed when you can look your shortcomings square in the eye and acknowledge them for what they are. That which you can change, you gently work towards changing, and that which you can't, you learn to love. No matter what card we are dealt, there is always one positive thing that can be reaped from the situation if you try your best to see beyond your eyes.

It's crucial to accept that you cannot accomplish everything. You must give yourself that leeway. Start to see how this facade of the strong black woman is hurting you. Accepting far too many responsibilities and saying "yes" far too frequently has a direct effect on how you feel about yourself.

When you get to the root of your need to constantly overachieve and soldier on despite feeling tired and exhausted by life, you find that this soldier mentality is fueled by a painful fact: you feel unloved, and so you constantly feel the need to prove your worth to others, so that they may finally love you. It's time to change that conception.

It's simple to forget to indulge in your favorite self-care activities, like unwinding with a nice movie or practicing meditation. Maybe instead of looking after someone else tonight, look after yourself. Perhaps you should indulge in a heartwarming bubble bath or take yourself out on a solo date. Although some of these self-love options may seem incredibly opulent, you need to set aside some time for yourself because you do so much every day. Ensure that you practice how to be with yourself, speak to yourself in a loving manner, and get to know yourself every day. We tend to assume that we know who we are since we spend time with ourselves all the time. However, if you don't try to spend more time with yourself and have an honest dialogue with yourself, you'll never come to know who you are, and thus, you will not be able to accept yourself in all of your beauty and flaws.

It's crucial to know when you need to rest. Knowing how to give yourself the grace to slow down and honor a crippling negative emotion is something that is considered to be the ultimate gesture of self-love. Trying to strike a balance between your professional life, social life, and relationships, puts us on a balance beam all the time. Often, your commute is the only opportunity you have to be alone.

I cannot stress enough how crucial it is to allow your head to remain calm and to feel at ease in that silence. Spend some time asking yourself, "Do I truly like my life? Do I enjoy what I have? Do I enjoy the thoughts and beliefs I have of myself?"

But doing that as a black woman can be quite challenging. Therefore, I strongly advise everyone to buy a journal or book and record their thoughts. Make a habit of doing this. Then, one year from now, read through your own writing. Don't read it the next day; wait a month and see how you feel about it. That will truly highlight where your real head is. Grab a journal, and then do the following:

- Start by analyzing the source of these emotions.
- Ask yourself: Where did I learn to put the needs of others above my own? Give it some thought. Why do I feel I need to defend the need for self-care?
- Apologize to yourself for pushing past your breaking point and failing to honor your need for self-love.

You could experience some sense of shame as you attempt to enhance your well-being. Black women frequently go through this. Society often gives us the impression that unless we toil assiduously to obtain them, the nice things that come to us are not something we deserve. We are taught to ignore symptoms of anxiety and despair in order to take care of everyone else, pushing through negative emotions. Consequently, you feel bad when you prioritize your health over others. It's time to let go of your guilt over engaging in radical self-love in order to improve your health.

It becomes difficult to ignore the indications urging you to take some time for yourself once you start to include it in your regular routine. For instance, if daily affirmations become a habit, you'll find yourself repeating them whenever you glance in the mirror. If Self-Love Sundays are a thing, then that calming walk to the park or that long bubble bath in the evening will feel as natural as brushing your teeth every morning. If questioning the nature of your negative thoughts is something you often do, then stopping to ask yourself why you have said something so unkind to yourself at that moment will be able to grant you more insight into ideas that may not even be yours to begin with. Some of these things are easier than others, and you won't magically become a self-love guru overnight. But that is why it is a journey and a beautiful one at that. Self-love will eventually become one of your healthiest habits if you start making it a ritual.

Start Where You Are

There is nothing more accurate than the saying, "comparison can be the thief of joy," especially in the context of self-love. The truth is that everyone starts from vastly different places on their journey of self-acceptance and love. Building one's self-worth and self-esteem will look quite different for every black woman, as we all have wounds in different places. However, every single journey only starts with a beginning, and a self-love and emotional healing journey for black women have a few things in common.

We are typically our own worst critics, as the cliché goes. By moving past that outdated maxim and establishing an environment where you may learn from your mistakes and grow, you can demonstrate self-love. Self-love is a wonderful aim to have, but it can be difficult to fulfill in practice, especially if you don't have a self-care routine. Self-care is a habit that, with time, can help you develop greater self-love. Even if you come from a place of self-hatred, harsh criticism, and perfectionism, it won't happen for you overnight. Still, you can gradually incorporate self-love into your life by consistently taking care of yourself. Your self-kindness, self-love, and sense of humanity will grow as a result of incorporating self-love practices into your daily routine in small, doable steps.

Accepting and Recognizing Your Emotional State

Nobody is content all of the time. People aren't constantly optimistic or being their best selves 24/7, despite what the highlight reels of social media may suggest. The ability to hold yourself to realistic standards is a crucial component of self-love. It's important to accept that some days are going to be better than others and that it's entirely normal to experience a bad day, a bad week, or even a bad season. In order to identify your emotions and learn to accept them, it's critical to frequently check in with your emotional state. In actuality, this means that you shouldn't act as though everything is alright when you know it's not.

This may sound counter-intuitive to ameliorating your well-being, but it actually relieves black women from the harmful burden of the strong black women trope. Being more candid about your feelings, firstly to yourself and then to others, will liberate you from needing to be a superwoman and accept that you are just a woman who sometimes needs a break and a breather. No matter where you are on your journey toward self-acceptance, this notion rings true. Black women need to learn how to gently acknowledge their pain without allowing it to consume them and learn how to sit with it to find out what truth it seeks to reveal.

You need to accept your emotional state in addition to acknowledging it. Adapting your plans or routine to your current state is a crucial component of accepting your feelings as they are. Any effective self-care regimen starts with learning to tune in to your emotional condition. It's also critical to know when a slump has lasted too long. While it's good to give yourself some leeway, take a break, or completely give in to a poor mood in certain circumstances, it's also critical to realize that our behaviors, routines, and habits can actually affect how we feel. If you are going through a serious rut, think about how you may improve your routine to try to get back into the groove. Self-care frequently involves striking a balance between being nice and forgiving to oneself and upholding positive coping mechanisms.

Take Time for Yourself

As enjoyable as it is to interact with others and socialize, it's crucial to set aside some time for yourself in order for you to assess your emotional state, the significance of which we discussed above, and spend some time taking care of yourself. Many people have the propensity to overextend themselves between jobs, everyday responsibilities, and social activities. And we understand that looking forward to a nice social occasion may frequently help people get through the week.

Who doesn't enjoy a solid Wednesday night plan that is refreshing enough to get them through the workweek? However, it's crucial that these social gatherings don't obstruct your essential alone time. Extreme FOMO sufferers may find it very challenging to decline a great movie with friends. However, sometimes engaging in activities that you generally find enjoyable leaves you feeling absolutely spent because you really need to have used that spare time to ponder and take care of yourself. Not that you should skip out on your social commitments, but you should schedule some time to engage in activities that will make you feel more alive. This can actually mean blocking out time on your to-do list to allow for rest.

Avoid aimlessly looking through your cellular device or watching TV during time set aside for self-care. Spend some time engaging in mindfulness exercises and other emotional awareness techniques. This can entail enrolling in a yoga class once a week, making plans to go for a walk, meditating, or starting a journal. As long as you're engaging in activities that relieve stress and make you feel grounded, there is no incorrect method to exercise self-care. Prioritizing your alone time in order for you to concentrate on self-love is not being selfish; it is an essential part of your self-care regimen.

Use Self-Talk

Learning to use constructive self-talk is a crucial step on the path to better self-care. Self-talk is the internal discourse that permeates our minds throughout the majority of the day. Self-talk is typically something we do subconsciously and is frequently a sign of our deepest sentiments and ideas. Self-talk can be highly negative at times, which can result in feelings of self-doubt, self-judgment, and even self-loathing. You can utilize mindfulness techniques to change your inner dialogue to a more positive one if you discover that your self-talk is disproportionately negative.

Giving positive affirmations to yourself is a simple and practical technique to achieve this. What aspects of yourself do you like? What do you take pride in? A regular reminder of these things can help you feel more upbeat and naturally inspire positive self-talk. You could do this as part of your mornings while brushing your teeth, for example. Recognizing when you are using negative self-talk is a crucial step in utilizing self-talk to your advantage. If you see this, try to identify the reason why, and then proceed in a forgiving manner that promotes optimism.

Overcoming a Self-Defeating Narrative

When we engage in negative self-talk for an extended period of time, we might begin to form negative stories about ourselves that can be seriously detrimental to our self-esteem. These self-deprecating stories wind up being internalized by us, and before we know it, they change our mindset and our behaviors.

You must recognize the unfavorable self-stories you are telling yourself in order to address the root of the issue. Where do these unfavorable rumors originate? Do they stem from a specific incident? The next step is to discover why you continue to believe these negative stories. You can help stop the toxic thought cycle that feeds negative self-talk if you can figure out why you keep telling yourself these stories. You can use the same constructive self-talk techniques outlined above to counter these negative stories. As a counter-attack, start offering your inner self-praise every time you can identify a negative self-talk pattern. Over time, you will be able to slowly change your inner dialogue.

Forgiveness of Oneself

To do this, practice self-compassion. We all make errors, no matter how big or small, and even while they may feel life-changing at the time, they probably aren't. Forgiveness is the glue that keeps life moving forward. The ability to reflect on your acts with love, understanding, and support when you embrace self-compassion will enable you to extend a forgiving hand to yourself for whatever transpired. It can be just as harmful to harbor grudges toward oneself as it is against other people. Forgive yourself for the times you called your hair ugly because it was natural. Forgive yourself for the times you walked in a room filled with Eurocentric-featured women and immediately felt small.

Forgive yourself for latching on to your intellect as a protective mechanism against the insufficiencies of feeling and being black. Forgive yourself for believing the lies. It can be really draining to hold onto a lot of negative energy when you have a grudge. By forgiving yourself and others, you can unshackle your energy and emotional storage to engage in more compassionate and loving behaviors. This will help you let go of any bad feelings you may have about yourself or your acts.

Committing to Loving Oneself

Being able to love oneself can take time; it does not happen suddenly. The poor habits we develop along the road that make us cruel to ourselves might be challenging to break. It's critical to keep in mind that this process can require dedication and time. Self-love is not about getting what you want right now. Whether it's buying a cute new shirt, indulging yourself in ice cream, or binge-watching a few episodes of your favorite show, most people are aware of how to cheer themselves up. They are enjoyable, and you should definitely keep doing them, but they are not sustainable paths to self-kindness and self-love. True self-love is founded in acceptance. Wake up every day, and make a pledge toward loving the totality of who you are, despite your insufficiencies, unfulfilled dreams, and failures.

Make a Commitment to Learn More

Nowadays, it seems like self-care and mindfulness are buzzwords, which is excellent because it means that everyone and especially black women, are learning to be more self-aware and accepting of who they are. Because of how recent this tendency is, new studies and methods are constantly being published. Trying new self-care methods and being informed as these concepts develop should be a key component of your self-care journey. We can always improve our ability to love and care for ourselves. Keeping up with the most recent research in the field might help you come up with original new ways to take care of yourself.

Failure is not Forever

If there is one thing that black women understand very well is how to fall and then get back up. If we are fortunate enough to be able to walk, which is a given for most of us, we experienced this precise and wonderful event when we were children. We've also experienced it numerous times in a metaphorical way as we navigate life's ups and downs. The real question is whether or not we will have the courage to get back up after falling.

Just keep in mind that mistakes are an acceptable part of being a human being, and they do not alter your value simply because you make them. Strength isn't being infallible, it is about having the fortitude and commitment to get back up after falling, despite our fear or doubt. We regain control over events, circumstances, and results in our lives by learning to see problems as opportunities. We gain valuable insight into what and who we really are and how to achieve success and contentment in a conscious, purposeful, and true manner when we can appreciate challenges, learn from them, and use them to our benefit. Living audaciously, pursuing our goals, and being ourselves in no way guarantees that we won't struggle, fail, or fall short. It's probably a good sign that we aren't playing all that large in our life if we aren't failing or encountering any problems at all.

Failure is a component of success, not its antithesis. It instructs us on resiliency, bravery, development, and support. Failure is a necessary step in the direction of all of our objectives. There is a 100% likelihood that every failure you experience will help you learn something. It is crucial to utilize failure as a learning tool to develop your character and your abilities, whether they are related to making decisions, solving problems, or anything else. Failure is often viewed as a sign of defeat, but you must modify this perception. We succeed, leave our comfort zone, and get fresh perspectives by learning from our mistakes and evolving from them.

From the time we take that first step till the present, failure is a constant in life. It makes us stronger and helps us develop. It also enables us to improve our strengths and learn from our flaws. Everybody makes mistakes, and every person handles failure differently. We must accept the likelihood that we will frequently stumble while traveling. But when we make the decision to get back up, pick ourselves up, be honest about how we're feeling and what occurred, and not allow it to hinder us from blossoming into who we were meant to be, we unlock the actual potential of strength, boldness, and authenticity.

Chapter 8: Build Your Self-Worth

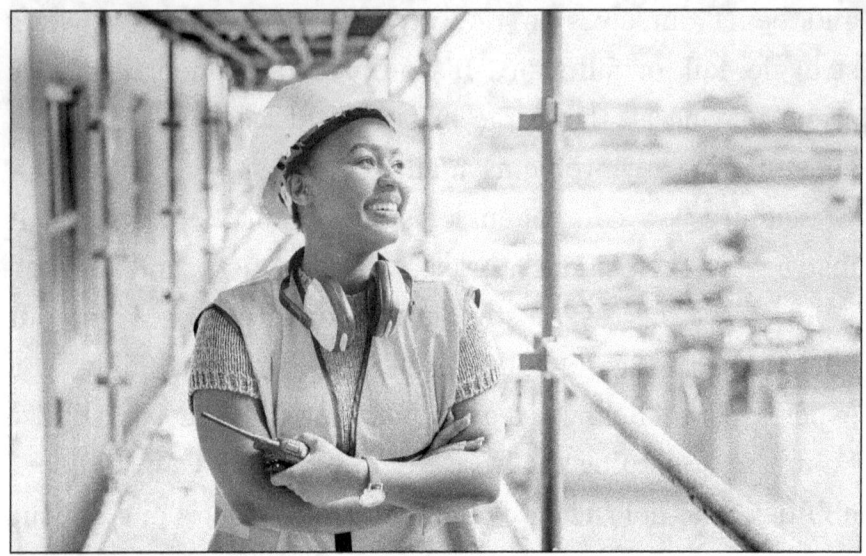

Although they are connected, self-esteem and self-worth differ significantly. Self-esteem refers to how you perceive and feel about yourself, and it can vary depending on your state of mind, your environment, your actions, and other people's opinions. Self-worth, which results from understanding and having a solid belief in your inherent value as a person, is a more comprehensive and steady kind of self-esteem. The things that you feel and think about yourself are characterized by self-esteem. Typically, it is based on assessments you have about yourself at the time. People who have low self-esteem lack self-assurance and tend to think and feel negatively about themselves more frequently. Low self-esteem can be temporary or persistent, with the latter more likely to result in emotional and behavioral issues. Self-esteem is unstable and inconsistent since it depends on how you feel about yourself and how confident you are. Instead, it mainly relies on the things, people, and external data you use to judge, compare, and evaluate yourself in the outside world.

Researchers define self-worth as a more inclusive, stable version of self-esteem that is unaffected by either internal or external variables. Self-worth refers to your fundamental views about your value and worth rather than focusing on particular characteristics, abilities, situations, or accomplishments. Self-worth isn't as likely to alter in response to feelings, attitudes, behaviors, or experiences because core beliefs are more likely to remain constant throughout time. High self-worth is seen to result in a more consistent and healthy form of self-esteem. It makes a person happier, healthier, and more successful in life while also offering defense against stress and emotional issues.

Healing the Inner Child

It is when you are a child that you begin to learn your first notions of self-worth. The loving embrace of a parent when you are irritated and in need of comfort tells the child that they are worthy of being loved even when they are in distress. A hug from a stranger who is soon to become a friend on the school playground tells the child that they are worthy of being a companion. The anatomy of childhood is where human beings learn and establish their most fundamental beliefs about their self-worth.

You may be familiar with the phrase "healing the inner child." Every adult has an inner child. It's that teeny, tiny portion of you that simply never matured.

Sometimes, this lack of maturity has been stifled by trauma, so there comes a need to heal the inner child. Events that occur when a person is young can have a lasting impact on their mind. The inner child can be wounded by a childhood friend moving away, physical or emotional abuse, or a damaged family. You might believe that the pain has passed. The subsequent pain, though, will live inside of you for the rest of your days, and it can occasionally rear its head when it's triggered by something. Inner child work is crucial on your path to developing self-trust as well as your overall trauma-healing journey. Because it was your younger self who first learned that you are unworthy, inadequate, and worthless. Therefore, if you desire to unlearn all the nonsense you were told about who you are, you need to involve the part of yourself that originally acquired it: your inner child.

Even while this type of emotional work is crucial for everyone, black women are especially in need of it. But it's challenging since black women are more likely to be the home breadwinners and single parents. Furthermore, taking time for oneself can seem selfish when you're carrying the responsibility of having to take care of everything, oftentimes alone.

Black girls undergo a series of discriminatory and alienating feelings when they grow up. One of the most insidious and yet less spoken of experiences is the adultification of little black girls. Adultification prejudice refers to how society perceives black girls as being less innocent and in need of protection than white girls.

There is a direct correlation between how society treats young black girls and its perception of black women as autonomous and strong. When black girls are adultified, they frequently develop into being less vocal about problems that are important to them since they are raised with no one listening to them. Little black girls were less able to ask for assistance when they needed it because they had been instructed to suck it up and figure things out on their own. They were instructed to concentrate on "more essential things," thus they were less able to tap into their emotions and less assured in their abilities as a result of being overlooked or rejected. . It is evident that a lot of the problems many adult black women experienced are caused by trauma they experienced as children. And so, one of the ways that black women can start to build their self-worth is through the healing of their inner child.

Realize the Problem

Recognizing that there is pain inside you and seeking to find out where it originates is the first step in healing. This can be the result of experiences you had as a child with adultification or racial prejudice in your family. Examine the connections between your adult habits and childhood difficulties like abandonment or trust.

Discover and Reinvent Who You Are

This exercise is crucial because it provides you the time to consider your future self, what matters to you, and how to break free from the labels that have been placed on you. In order to learn more about oneself, you can ponder the following questions:

- What do you like to do?
- Which kind of life do you envision for yourself?
- What principles do you want to uphold?
- How can you make room in your life for greater creativity?

Write Yourself a Letter

Writing a letter to the little black girl you once were is a strategy that is frequently employed in therapy. By doing this, you may be able to forgive yourself and others, as well as heal old wounds and find closure. What to include in a letter to yourself:

- Select the age or time period you wish to concentrate on.
- Be honest and approach this letter with kindness. Write to your child as though you were a devoted parent.
- As a child, tell yourself the things you wish you had been told.
- Utilize this letter to explain the situation, offer a different viewpoint, and reassure yourself when you were younger.
- Write on till you experience a feeling of relief.
- You are free to reread it and take any action you like.

Practice Radical Self-Care

Although self-care has received a lot of attention lately, each person must define it for themselves based on their own

requirements. Here are some methods for engaging in radical self-care:
- Establish clear boundaries.
- Make a nighttime and a morning routine.
- Pay attention to your gut feelings.
- Enjoy being by yourself.
- Put your own happiness first.

Give Yourself What You Lacked as a Child

Because you couldn't defend yourself or speak up in certain circumstances as a child, you might have felt powerless. You have the opportunity to give yourself, as an adult, what you wished your parents or caregivers would have done for you. This could involve financial or psychological gifts.

Embracing My Blackness

According to a 2019 Pew Research Center survey, over 75% of black adults say that being black has a significant impact on how they view themselves, either highly (52%) or very (22%). Comparatively, approximately six out of ten persons who identify as Hispanic (59%) and 56% of adults who identify as Asian (56%) agree that being either of those identities is very important to who they are. Only 15% of white adults view race as being fundamental to who they are. The proportion of black adults who identify primarily via their race fluctuates with age; those under the age of 30 place less importance on race than those over the age of 30. So, it is pretty evident that blackness is important to black people.

More often than not, experiencing the effects of one's blackness has a negative connotation attached to it. But on the journey towards building self-worth, black women need to find a way to re-configure that narrative so that their identification with blackness begins to carry a positive connotation to it as well. This is how that fundamental notion of self-worth gets replaced by something stronger and more powerful. Let us take the example of Brianna.

Although she has always known that black was beautiful, it wasn't until recently that she truly understood how beautiful blackness truly is. She became aware of what it meant to be a young black girl growing up in a predominantly white society in elementary school when she attended school while residing in the little town of Kinston, North Carolina.

In the second grade, she was chosen to enroll in academically talented courses. She was the only black female in the class, along with a black boy with whom she is still friends with till this very day. She can recall instances when she felt timid because she thought nobody would or could understand her and she was alone. In an effort to blend in with her white peers and find acceptance and friendship, she suppressed who she was. Early on, her mother had to teach her how to develop a thick skin. Her mother believed it was crucial for her to forbid others from underestimating her abilities. Brianna had to develop her inner strength in solitude.

As she got older, she was more aware of her blackness, but it wasn't until she read Zora Neale Hurston's novel, *Their Eyes Were Watching God* in high school that she understood the beauty of Janie's difficulties as a strong black woman.

When she started at the University of North Carolina, Chapel Hill, she had no idea that the book would aid her in creating her own path of becoming a black woman.

Brianna started college with four other black women who later became her dearest friends. They served as her primary source of encouragement and helped her accept her status as a black student at a primarily white college. Although they assisted her in navigating the complexities of a collegiate experience as a young black woman, Brianna only found herself truly starting to search for her own identity on November 25, 2014.

She vividly recalls that day because it was the fateful morning following Darren Wilson's complete acquittal on all charges related to shooting and killing unarmed black teen Michael Brown in Ferguson, Missouri.

That day was incredibly dismal and dark, reflecting how Brianna was feeling on the inside. It was the first time as a senior in her school that she felt invisible and undervalued. On that particular day, she took part in a nonviolent demonstration and "die-in" on campus, where students shared their firsthand accounts of police brutality while also sharing what it was like to be black in America. She felt as though she was in a dream. Brianna had the impression that she was getting a better understanding of what it was like to be an oppressed minority and not to be treated with the same respect as her non-black college counterparts.

Her perspective of the world significantly shifted at that precise instant. She became aware that she had, once again, become the main target of America due to something as trivial as her pigment and her gender.

After that particular protest, she made the decision to start her search for, and embrace, her identity as a 21-year-old black woman.

Brianna felt a profound remorse for the tragedy that led to her journey, but she became committed to learning about her blackness in America. She didn't know where to begin, but it made her feel better to know that, despite black people's disparate personal histories, she was part of a tribe that would support her along the road. Since black people were largely unified based on similar life challenges, she knew that there was a sense of companionship in going through the process together as a community.

Due to the fact that her institution is one of the oldest public universities in the country and was founded by slaves, she first took the time to read about the contributions that black people have made throughout history. The research period was highly illuminating and had a significant impact on how it shaped her identity. She started finding out about notable black individuals like George Moses Horton, a slave and the first African American to publish a book in the South. By studying African-American literature and completing African-American psychology courses, she was also able to obtain a deeper understanding of the beauty of her blackness.

Her experience continued while she pursued her journalism master's degree at the University of Maryland. Graduate school undoubtedly made her more aware and encouraged her to live a carefree black girl's life. She took the initiative to gain control of her education. She determined that the best way for her to give back to the world was to write about current events, particularly those that have an impact on the black community. She developed an interest in producing stories about the black experience to inform others about the importance of their ancestors to both their race and history.

Living in the Washington Metropolitan Area exposed Brianna to diversity, freedom of expression, and various nuances of blackness. The setting continues to provide her with the inspiration she requires to maintain her sense of self-worth and belief that she is capable of doing anything. She has found serenity in the knowledge that there is beauty in being black, despite the fact that she feels like identifying her blackness is a perpetual struggle. Her experiences have boosted her self-esteem and helped her build a sense of pride in herself. What she is most proud of is that she now has a greater grasp of who she truly is as a black woman residing in America.

Her journey has been difficult, but she has reached a place where she understands who she is as a human being, and she is eager to see who she will develop into in the future. Most significantly, Brianna has discovered that while no two people's identities are identical, their shared African heritage unites them despite their differences.

Briana is now pursuing a profession as a writer for black media, at the age of 25 to celebrate the diversity and unending beauty of blackness. By promoting black pride, black love, and being unapologetically black through shared experiences, black people stand the chance to realize that their blackness is a gift.

With time, Brianna has learned to accept her full lips, her melanin-filled skin, and her 4C gravity-defying hair. These characteristics have taught her how important it is to be different and free.

Brianna is one story of many black women who began to fight against the racial narratives that sought to suppress and oppress them. If you log on to any social media platform, you will find the unhindered celebration of black beauty in all its glory. This is tremendously important, particularly for black women who were told that they were ugly and bottom of the barrel for most of their lives. Black women are now carving out the space to validate themselves and praise their accomplishments, and features, while simultaneously healing the wounds of that little black girl who felt unprotected and unloved. These are the black women that will have daughters who know their self-worth, not only because they are black and beautiful, but because the element of divinity that resides in every single human being is lodged in their spirit too.

I am More Than Just a Black Woman

While there is undeniable power in building your self-worth as a black woman by embracing all of the beauty of blackness in a world that vehemently wants you to believe otherwise, there is also the value that comes from seeing yourself as more than the black woman. First and foremost, before all of these injurious and divisive tribal labels were placed on us, we are human beings, and all human beings require the same things, belonging, meaning, and safety.

Black women have become the poster children of black activism. More often than not, when you think about Black Lives Matter, a picture of a black lady holding a placard comes to mind. Few people, however, are willing to discuss the psychological consequences of making your entire life about eradicating social injustice.

While it's a great idea to pay attention to how the world oppresses you as a black woman, the truth is that this type of information is heavy. It will eventually become a problematic burden to carry continuously. For one thing, spending too much time focusing on all the wrongs in the world is simply not healthy for anyone. Focus on acting in practical ways that will actually have an impact on the community rather than allowing yourself to become deeply enmeshed in the Black Lives Matter movement to the point that you cannot find an identity beyond being black.

Supporting black female entrepreneurs and businesses that enhance and advance the image of black women is one example of being a staunch supporter of black success without needing to carry the weight of its difficulties on your shoulder. Support media representations of black women as valued, deserving of protection, and deserving of respect. Stream the songs of darker-skinned black women in media, and buy products from businesses run by black women. Consistently showing support to your community should be a priority, particularly if you are a more sensitive woman and easily predisposed to feelings of anxiety and depression.

This is not to say that black women shouldn't be activists. In fact, it is black women's undeniable activism since the era of slavery that has led to some of the most important liberations in history. Activism is vital for black people, and it will not stop being so until black people achieve the complete freedom that they deserve. However, finding ways to base your identity on other facets of your life can prove to be as beneficial to the psychological well-being of black women. If you work in activism, and dealing with issues plaguing black women is your full-time job, then you could benefit from having hobbies or other external realities that you can equally rely on for a sense of identity. You are not just a black woman, you are also a professional, you are a mother, a daughter, a sister, a dancer, a reader, a musician, an athletic person, a Christian, a Muslim, a dog lover, a cat lover, a foodie, a quirky girl. You are a human being with a complex nature and complex interests.

Having a sense of identity that is nestled into many things is one of the healthiest ways that a black woman can come to appreciate all of the things that truly make her a valuable and complex human being. Every other race is allowed to find their identities in their pursuits and realities, so black women should feel comfortable enough to do the same. This type of conceptualization allows your emotional well-being to remain robust as you gather positive energy from the progress that you make across various domains and will enable that progress to fuel you and make you truly feel like you are continuously growing and progressing as a full entity, and not just as a portion of yourself, which is being a black woman.

Chapter 9: Prioritize Your Goals

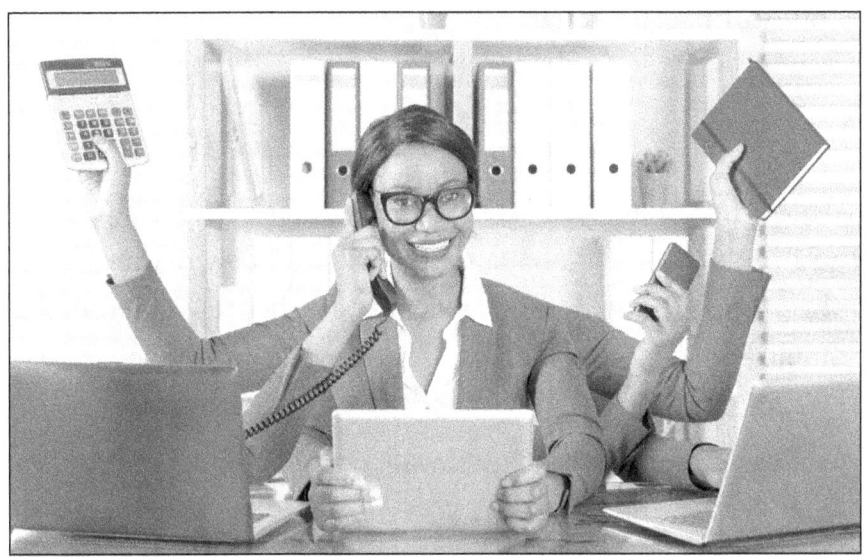

The practice of categorizing your goals according to their importance, value, and urgency is known as goal prioritization. You must also allocate your energy, time, and resources where they are most needed during this process. It's really just a fancy way of saying what you are probably already doing: prioritizing what needs to be done first before tackling other activities.

Prioritizing your goals means tackling everything on your to-do list while beginning the day with what matters most. Why wouldn't you want to exert the most effort toward the objectives that have the potential to yield the highest return on investment? You do, and goal prioritizing can help you locate these goals and plan how to reach them.

Prioritizing goals can reduce stress and increase productivity. Since it enables you to allocate your time among your objectives, it can also enhance your time management abilities. This leads to an overall improved emotional health profile for black women.

Let Go of Regrets

While A huge part of being able to set goals in the first place is the beliefs we have about them, without belief, there is no movement, and a lot of our positive beliefs can only be established once we let go of the regrets we have accrued throughout the years.

Regret. The one who got away, or the job opportunity you didn't accept, the argument you wish you hadn't gotten into, the decision made to go to the incorrect school, the investment you didn't make, the money you didn't save, the move you wish you'd made, and on and on and on. It seems to be a reality of life. Life is predictable in that manner; there will undoubtedly be some decisions you make along the way that you wish you had made differently. Regrets can be major; such as choosing a career that doesn't suit your goals or minor such as choosing a dress for a wedding that you truly don't feel confident wearing. You may experience everyday regrets or overarching regrets that simply appear to influence everything you do.

Regret by itself is not harmful; in fact, it might motivate us to take positive action. An advertisement or a parent playing carefreely at the playground with their child of a similar age may be seen by the parent who has been working too much and maybe distracted around the kids. This parent might have a fleeting sorrow about not focusing more on their own child, and they might then choose to spend more time with them.

Once they learn they have a fatal illness, some people feel guilty about the time they have squandered and decide to make the most of every moment they have left. When approaching retirement age, someone who later decides they made the wrong professional decision may choose to leave their current position and start their dream job. There are countless examples of people who were inspired by remorse and changed their direction, tried something new, or followed a different path.

However, regret can become an albatross for some people. Believing that you never make the right decisions or that you always choose the wrong thing for yourself can often result in having too many regrets. Remorse can also paralyze you because it makes you regret what you should or could have done and prevents you from moving on with better decisions. It starts to feel akin to speeding down the highway while continually scanning your rear-view mirror for things you've left behind. Driving without paying attention to what's ahead of you and what's in front and beside you is risky, not to mention that you don't get to appreciate the beauty of the view as you pass it.

It could be time to let go of the regretted decision and find a way to courageously move on to a new phase of your life. The only thing a person has at their disposal to work with is their current state, and ideally, their future state, even though you can learn from every error you make along the way. The real action takes place in the present; thus, your commitment should be in the now and resolve to make better judgments in the future.

But how can you divert your focus if it has become firmly fixed on the rearview mirror? Consider taking the following actions to stop looking behind and start focusing on the now and your future:

Own It

Indeed, whatever occurred did occur. You made the incorrect decision, said the wrong thing, and moved on the incorrect path. It's finished, whatever it was. It is done. You won't always make intelligent decisions or decisions that are tilted towards the actualization of your best interests because that is a truth of life. There are occasions when you lack the necessary knowledge. Sometimes thinking prevails over emotions, and other times your "gut" takes precedence. You might not be able to carve out enough time to go through all of the options at your disposal and could feel under pressure to make a decision. Whatever the situation may be, the fact remains that not everyone is always in a position to make the best choice possible. You need to find ways to extend some grace to yourself and accept that whatever you did at that time, no matter how ineffective it was or terrible the outcome of it ended up being, was done because you believed that it was the best possible option at the time. We live, and we learn.

Learn From It

Make an effort to assess what happened objectively. Why did you act in the manner that you did? This is not the time to criticize oneself; instead, it is the time to evaluate what happened. By attempting to truly comprehend what went wrong, you can discover a lot about your decision-making process. Is it the case that you need to acquire information more effectively the next time? Do you require extra time to consider something? Are other people influencing your decision-making process? Take note of what needs to be done differently when you are faced with the need to make a choice once again.

Describe What You Want in Writing

Focus on "what I want" rather than focusing on "what if I had" whether you regret a relationship that ended, a professional pathway that never came to fruition, a financial decision, or an educational experience. Although you cannot go back in time, you can focus on the present circumstances. So, this career isn't the greatest one for you; how do you describe what you do want? What should you do now that the person you were with for over seven years has left? How can you build a life for yourself as a single person? Since you weren't able to obtain the education of your dreams, how can you create a strategy to enroll in classes or get involved at the institution you did go to? Make the most out of what you already have while seeking to find ways to ameliorate it.

Carpe Diem

Pay attention to your senses. Increase your senses of smell, taste, hearing, and enjoyment while you are actively engaged in your daily tasks. Get involved with your surroundings. Make a commitment to being present with what is happening and pay attention to things you haven't noticed previously. Life is now; whatever occurred to you in the past has no control over this present reality. Engage in the present and sharpen your awareness of your surroundings. You won't be able to concentrate on your regrets in the rearview mirror if you divert your field of attention to what is standing right before your eyes, as the mind cannot focus on two things at once.

Plan an Action That Might Assist in Offsetting Your Regrets

For instance, your children may not visit you as often today because you did not spend enough time with them while they were young. Consider helping out at a children's home or signing up for a program. Perhaps the issue is that you were unable to pursue the career path that you always wanted. Instead of feeling sorry for yourself, you could pick up aspects of that career and create a hobby from it instead. Life is not a straight line, nor is it a binary world. What nuances of gray may you add to your life, even if they don't necessarily eradicate your regret, could find a way to give your life a different sense of meaning.

Fight for What You Believe and Stop Living for Others

If there's one thing that black women have done incessantly throughout history, it is to live for others. Taking back the space that you need to thrive in your body is one of the most fundamental steps toward emotional health.

The biggest thing standing between people and their dreams is their opposing beliefs. What's holding you back, you must wonder, if you feel like an undiscovered genius trapped in the day-to-day laboriousness of a dead-end job? It's probably your unfavorable beliefs holding you back from going after that which you believe you were truly meant to do. Our beliefs are formed mainly by the messages we've been exposed to when we were little. For instance, your parents may have informed you that no one in the family has been successful at generating income or true wealth. Your brain sucks this information up like a sponge and deep into your subconscious mind, and you become more inclined to accept this message as true the more times you hear it.

Because you've convinced yourself that trying to generate money is futile, you'll avoid endeavors that could result in financial success, such as learning more about investment strategies or completing an MBA. This aspect of your character prevents you from pursuing your dreams. Fortunately, you are certainly capable of overcoming this erroneously paralyzing information. How? by forming optimistic thoughts that give you confidence in yourself. Start by observing and analyzing who you truly are as though you were a complete stranger. Be proud of your accomplishments and consider all the positive things you can say about yourself. Allow your cells to swell up with pride regarding all the amazing things you have done in this lifetime that you may not have even thought to congratulate yourself for.

Generate some empowering beliefs out of these reflections. Negative attitudes that you've carried in your psyche for so long only serve the purpose of holding you back if you start to feel like you're talented, that your ideas are meaningful, and that you have something to contribute to the world. This is when the true transformative journey officially starts. Don't let other people tell you to give up; instead, figure out who you want to be. We have an innate sense of understanding who we are and how we behave when we are young. But as we become older, we stop trusting our inner guidance and start following what other people urge us to do.

You must embrace your inner beast if you want to achieve your goals. You can choose your own route once you stop caring what other people think. Do you aspire to be an author? Then knowing that you will need to clock in a solid number of hours writing to achieve this should transmute from a daunting contemplation to something that awakens a deep sense of passion in you. But there will be sacrifices that will come along your way. You will probably need to find time to relax while maintaining work that allows you to pay your rent. Your "hobby" may make your coworkers laugh. As you spend more time working on your novel and less time with friends, they may fade away. These adjustments can be painful, but perseverance is required if you desire to truly become a published author.

You'll have the fortitude to overlook other people's condemnation if you recognize how admirable it is that you are following your own path. Granted, finding your calling isn't always simple.

The requirements or responsibilities of family and friends encircle many of us. But if you choose a profession like a doctor or a lawyer simply because it's in your family's bloodline, you'll end up detesting your work and your decisions. So pay attention to your gut feeling and take some time to examine your lifestyle, your activities, and your actual areas of interest. You'll be able to determine what you genuinely desire from life by reflecting in this way.

For a richer, happier life, you have to harbor an abundant willingness to learn, practice appreciation, and master forgiveness. Make the most of your brief time here on earth by living fully. Though it's all too easy to overlook this in the hustle culture of modern living, each day is an opportunity to appreciate and celebrate life's journey. There is no greater joy than truly pursuing your purpose, especially when you have spent years feeling like the world wanted nothing to do with you.

Think of yourself as a voracious learner. People who are passionate about learning don't feel under pressure to demonstrate their skills, so they don't struggle with the commonly crippling fear of failing either. Making mistakes is no longer a terrifying black woman but rather a welcome step in the learning process. Imagine that you are a competitive ice skater. Every loss and setback to your self-esteem can feel like failure if you view yourself as a champion. Instead, if you approach new difficulties with a lighthearted attitude and greater bravery to take the necessary risks that have the ability to push you to learn more, you'll find yourself becoming a lifelong learner of life.

Make the daily effort to feel and express your gratitude for being alive. Being grateful is a condition of being; it's not about expressing gratitude, only to be polite. Being thankful forces all the positive aspects of life to remain at the forefront of your mind. Additionally, by cultivating and expressing thankfulness, you might encourage others to do the same. Let's take the example of a close-knit team at work. By concentrating on the accomplishments of your team, you inevitably practice gratitude. Perhaps you are grateful for your ability to maintain openness, honesty, and kindness in your conversation. Or your team works hard to control their egos. Maybe your work culture is positive and accommodating for a black woman. Be grateful for whatever it is!

In the modern world, being action-oriented and a go-getter is one of the most praised skill sets. On the other hand, we don't frequently establish the habits of thinking things through and giving ourselves time to develop ideas before we take action, even though we should. Maybe you want to be a writer, but you're not sure how to get your work published. One of the things you could do instead of just jumping straight into writing is doing some research on authors that inspired you and investigated how they fulfilled their dreams to get inspiration for your own journey. Proper planning prevents poor performance.

However, actions build confidence in a way that planning cannot. Instead of contemplating extensively on the act, don't concentrate on your shaking hands or your hesitant voice if you want to become a good speaker but are uncomfortable speaking in front of a group of people.

Instead, picture yourself giving engaging talks, and you'll start to present with more assurance and expertise in no time. This is known as a virtuous circle: the more speeches you deliver, the more confident you get and the better your public speaking becomes.

In pursuing your goals, thought is a strong tool, but it must be used in conjunction with effective action. You must first go through the resistance of delaying and hesitancy in order to take effective action. When we put off making decisions, we allow our fear of failure to hold us back. You'll look for any excuse not to try anything if you believe you're unqualified to do it. Your progress will be impeded by beliefs like "My writing isn't good enough" or "I'll never be able to monetize my skills." Without diving in, you will simply never know how deep the ocean is.

You need to remind yourself of your goals in order to remove some of these self-defeating justifications. If your willpower is lacking, you might need to reevaluate your objectives. You must get past your hesitation in order to take action. We often hold back because we don't want to change into someone else that we or others might not like. Imagine that your goal is to perform on stage, capturing the admiration of crowds in a commanding presence. But when you give this goal some serious thought, you pause. After all, you've never been a fan of extroverts, and as far as you are concerned, the majority of people also have wrong opinions about them. Will working as an actor make you the person you despise? No. Simply learn to get through your doubts because on the other side of these feelings is a reality that can make you proud.

Take some time to reflect on complex topics like "Will it make me happy?" and "Do I truly want to be an actor?" It's time to identify your reluctance and procrastination for what they truly are. It is time to stop making excuses. In order to achieve your desired goal, you have decided to alter your course of action. How far are you willing to go? Talented individuals rarely achieve their goals because they quit too easily.

Keep in mind that rejection and failure are universal aspects of life. Both legendary basketball player Michael Jordan and film director Steven Spielberg were turned down several times. Even though everyone experiences rejection along the way, you should never give up. Instead, draw lessons from your experienced failures and continue to work hard until you get the life you've always desired. You must exercise responsibility in every area of your life if you want to resist the urge to give up. It's time to make some deliberate changes if your routines, environment, or friend groups make it tougher for you to accomplish your goals. There is no shame in going to that "white" school if you believe that it is the conduit to your ultimate career goal. There is no shame in doing what you know is necessary for your happiness and well-being.

In fact, one of the best ways to keep on track is to adopt new surroundings and ways of life that are focused on your life's mission. If you want to become a writer, hang out with people who share your interests. Make sure you begin and end your day in a way that constantly reminds you of your objectives.

Your newfound life will ultimately materialize via activity, strong desires, and clear objectives.

Give yourself the unconditional permission to pursue your aspirations and, more importantly, stop caring what other people think. Learn to identify the aspects of your life that prevent you from living for yourself, and then make adjustments to your way of thinking and living to remove these obstacles. Importantly, keep doing what you truly love, and don't allow anyone to pull you away from it! You'll soon find yourself leading the life you've always imagined.

You have been raped, used, and abused for centuries. This is your time to break free from all of the shackles, break free from the angry black woman. Break free from the strong black woman. Break free from the expectations of you being single or a baby mama. Break free from the expectations that you can do everything alone. Do what your soul has brought you here to do. That is the best antidote to the violence of this existence. Purpose.

We're not here to fulfill the dreams of others while ignoring our own, keeping them concealed and unspoken. We're not only here to exist for others; there's more to life than that. Making every minute count is the finest way to use our time while we are on this planet. That's acceptable if you're attempting to actualize the aspirations and objectives of other people. But if that's not how you want to spend your days, then it's time to start living for yourself.

Managing Expectations

Once again, bringing the strong black woman trope is critical in this conversation. The world has set unrealistic expectations for black women, and they have been desperately trying to meet this to the detriment of their emotional well-being.

Expectations can enslave black women in two different ways, making both your career and personal lives much harder than they need to be. Standards must be followed. However, there is a significant distinction between "expectations" and having agreed-upon metrics for behavior or performance. An expectation isn't an agreed-upon metric set among individuals; instead, expectations are convictions that a particular result or event will take place. Expectations are merely speculation about what something could bring and are founded on deeply held beliefs.

An Example of Expectations

A man's wife has a birthday on a given day, and he wishes to surprise her. To ensure that she would be pleasantly delighted by the surprise when she got home, he had planned everything he was certain she would adore. The lights were turned down, scented candles were lit, and he had made a delicious meal for her. Her favorite flowers were used in the centerpiece, and the music was just what he anticipated she would like. "Ugh," she exclaimed as she entered. My day has been terrible. Not even hungry, really. Going to take a bath now. She doesn't even acknowledge all of the efforts that her husband put into the evening. He is upset. How dare she? How dare she not be grateful for all that he has done?

Then he understood that she had fallen short of his expectations, but it wasn't her fault. She was under no responsibility to live up to his expectations; they were his. This story contains an important lesson that we should apply to all facets of our lives. Expectations do not guarantee outcomes, and more often than not, they only lead to hurt feelings and disappointments. The husband was at first disappointed that his wife didn't respond as he'd expected, and his wife was astonished and unhappy that he was displeased with her for only wishing she could take a long bath after a difficult day.

Expectations Can Shackle You in Two Ways

You can be bound by expectations in two different ways. When you create expectations of others, like in the case of the husband, you are engaging in the first form of expectation. The second is when other people place unrealistic expectations on you, which would be the case with the wife. A life skill that can help you as you navigate your day, from work to family and other things, is being aware of each of these potential hazards and, more importantly, how you can avoid them. You'll be amazed by how frequently expectations come into play throughout your day once you learn to detect them. When you realize that even the expectations you set for yourself are merely your best hypotheses shaped into theory, you will feel free from the tight shackle that you didn't even know you were in all along. Expectations are simply predictions and, essentially, our firmly held beliefs flavored with a healthy dose of hope. Unfortunately, letting go of them can prove to be harder than we think, but we can engage in practices that help us acknowledge an expectation for what it is and rid ourselves of the guilt and shame that we experienced as a result of an unmet expectation.

Three Ways to Prevent Setting Unrealistic Expectations

Don't ever assume: Ask if you're unsure. Ask yourself if this is truly what you want to do. Black women have had expectations imposed on them from a very young age. The odds are not in their favor, and their parents know this, so they expect their young daughters to become over-achievers. They expect their young daughters to pursue a career path for financial benefit and not for true passion. All of these things are expected of you, but don't assume that you want them simply because it is so. Learn to listen to your own inner voice.

Recognize that eliminating expectations from your interactions, both professional and personal, is not only smart but also compassionate: It is never pleasant to be misunderstood. Even the most reclusive person among us humans actually thrives when we have a sense of connection to others. When assumptions are made about others, and those assumptions turn out to be incorrect, the results can be very unpleasant since those people may feel that they haven't lived up to expectations. Disengaging yourself from an expectation that was set for you is not problematic; it is compassionate.

Enjoy the way your life is right now: We tend to compare our lives with that of others far too frequently and always fall short in some way. Then add in those illusions and desires that are really just expectations disguised as fantasies, such as "I'll be happier when I get a promotion at my job," or "when we are married, I'll finally be happy," and so on and so forth. It is crucial that you enjoy the day right before you. Avoid confusing expectations with goals. Goals almost always guide you, while expectations almost always leave you disappointed.

Set Realistic Expectations

Although the ideal would be to not set expectations of yourself at all, it can be difficult and almost nearly impossible to do so. The next best thing, then, would be to set realistic expectations of yourself.

When we have unrealistic expectations, we expect that we will work nonstop. Every day, we anticipate having the same amount of high energy and functionality. We expect that we will feel the same feelings, calm, and contentment with ourselves. We anticipate that we will be fearless. We even expect that we will have the ability to handle difficult moments like a to-do list. We'll deal with our melancholy with ease and strength and just as we would with email or a kitchen cleanup session. These unrealistic expectations can cause us not only burnout physically but emotionally as well. It's impossible to always be able to show up with vitality and energy every single day, especially as women. We have a cycle and hormonal fluctuations during the month that leave us lethargic and, in some cases, even depressed. We need to be able to honor that reality without feeling like constant machines. We need to be realistic about our expectations so that we may thrive even in the face of a storm.

Analyze Your Expectations

Ask yourself what the past has demonstrated to you regarding your expectations: Has it ever been successful? Has it evolved over time? What causes this expectation and the worry that you won't fit in with the crowd? Would you still have this expectation of yourself if you didn't care what other people thought of you? Do you really think you can achieve your goal given the hours in your day, the people you have in your life, and the time you have available? Ask yourself these questions.

Silence Your Fear

Fear frequently gives rise to irrational expectations. We don't even realize how much fear we carry around with us in our bodies. An excellent way to manage fear in the short term is to practice taking slow deep breaths for three to five minutes per day, twice a day. Pay attention to the areas of your body where tension is held. When other thoughts come to mind, focus on your breathing. This teaches the body to invite calmness and openness rather than making choices and setting expectations based on fear.

Investigate Your Feelings of Inadequacy

Unrealistic aspirations result from the fundamental conviction that we are insufficient. When we live here, we never really live with the purpose of enjoying the totality of our existence; instead, we live in regret over what we aren't, and anxiety over what we might never be. Coming to the realization that this is not an innate belief can help us begin to disprove it. Most of the inadequacy felt by black women is a result of the unfair societal prison that they have been placed in. Before accepting a self-defeating and injurious expectation as a truth, investigate it further to get to the origins of its conception.

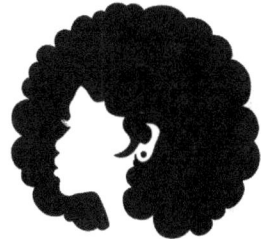

Conclusion

The black woman has been wounded by society, and today she finds herself having to conform to detrimental notions that leave her overworked and undervalued, further perpetuating a toxic cycle. The black woman has been violated and abandoned. She has been made to feel inferior to every other human being, and her self-worth has been run through the mud. The black woman was never protected, and she knows this. The effects of an oppressive reality run through her stride. They are in the callouses of her hands and in the uncertainty of her smile. Her fight is lodged in the bags under her sleepless eyes and in the educated choice of her words. The black woman is strong, yes, but the black woman needs to heal. And so, she must unlearn all of the things that she has learned.

The black woman needs to combust in the fire of her own doing. She needs to incinerate the racialized ideals of the strong black woman, of the angry black woman, and of the jezebel that the world so desperately wants to see her become. The black woman must burn these oppressive notions in a violent fire and emerge again from the ashes, like a phoenix, brand new. The black woman needs to rise with feathers of hope. She needs to come back as the human black woman, the one that is unafraid to claim the rest that she needs. She needs to come back as the assertive black woman, the one that states her business without fear of what the world may say. She needs to come back as the woman, the one who is valued and seen as more than what lies between her legs.

The black woman has a long journey toward restoring her humanness and allowing her inner world to heal, but black woman, we can do this together.

We believed that we needed to become like men to survive in their world, and though it may have served us to a point, we are tired and in need of a home. Let us create that home for each other. Let us nurture each other. Cry with each other and heal each other. Let us learn what it truly means to be women. Let us allow ourselves the privilege of fully being human. Let us heal. Let us rise.

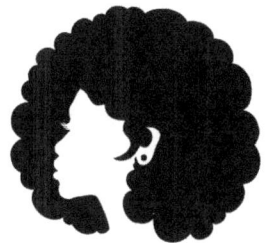

Thank You

Before you go, I just wanted to thank you for purchasing my book.

There are many books on the same topic, but you took a chance and chose this one.

So, thank you for choosing me and reading this book to the end.

Now, I wanted to ask you for a small favor: Could you please consider posting a review for the book? Reviews are the easiest way to support an independent author like me.

Your feedback will help me continue creating books that will help you achieve your desired results. So, if you enjoyed it, please let me know.

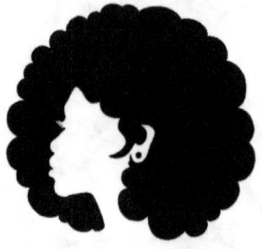